THE STATE OF YOUR MIND AND BODY

RELATIONSHIP BETWEEN THE BRAIN AND THE BODY

HERB LAWRENCE

CONTENTS

Chapter 1

RELATIONSHIP BETWEEN THE BRAIN AND THE BODY

Chapter 2

AGGRESSIVE MENTAL ATTITUDES

Chapter 3

CONSIDER YOUR MENTAL AND PHYSICAL WELL BEING

Chapter 4

IN TERMS OF BOTH YOUR MENTAL AND PHYSICAL HEALTH

Chapter 5

EXCESSIVE STRESS AND ANXIETY ABOUT THE FUTURE

Chapter 6

AFFECTIVE DISORDERS OR ANXIETY RELYING EXCESSIVELY ON ONE'S MEMORIES

Chapter 7

RAPID ADAPTATION TO PRESSURED CONDITIONS IS A HALLMARK OF STRESS

Chapter 8

INJURIES TO THE MIND

Chapter 9

FEELINGS OF GUILT AND THEIR ACHE

Chapter 10

CHANGE OF HEART AND HOPE

Chapter 1

RELATIONSHIP BETWEEN THE BRAIN AND THE BODY

There is no denying the connection between the brain and the rest of the body. The mind-body link is a concept that has been around since ancient times, when it was first discussed by philosophers. You don't have to be a philosopher to wonder if there's a connection between your mind and body.

Today, when we discuss the mind-body connection, we are talking to the ways in which one's physical health can either positively or negatively affect one's mental and emotional well-being. It is believed that if we keep a happy attitude and focus on helping others, our minds and bodies will work together like clockwork, while the opposite is true: that we will not be at our mental or emotional peak if our physical health is poor. It's common sense that when you're feeling down, it's difficult to be in a good mood, and vice versa when you're feeling up. In this post, we'll go over several self-care practices that can help you maintain a healthy mind and body.

The brain and body are connected by neural networks made up of neurotransmitters, hormones and chemicals. From breathing and digestion to pain perception and motor control to thought and emotion, our daily lives are orchestrated by signals traveling along these channels.

CHRONICLE OF THE RELATIONSHIP BETWEEN THE MIND AND BODY

The idea that the mind and body are inextricably linked is not new. In fact, up until around 300 years ago, nearly every medical system around the world addressed both. However, beginning in the 17th century, Westerners began to view the mind and body as separate. The body was seen as something akin to a machine, with parts that could be replaced and functioned independently of one another, and with no link to the consciousness.

This Western perspective was crucial in advancing allopathic fields including surgery, trauma treatment, and medications. However, it drastically diminished scientific exploration of the human emotional and spiritual life and undervalued people's intrinsic capacity to heal.

This viewpoint began to shift progressively in the twentieth century. After first dismissing the idea of a link between the brain and the rest of the body, scientists have recently begun to prove the existence of intricate connections between the two. "extensive research has proved the physiological and mental advantages of meditation, mindfulness training, yoga, and other mind-body activities," writes James Lake, MD, an integrative psychiatrist at Stanford University.

THE MIND BODY CONNECTION HOW DOES IT OPERATE

Your thoughts and beliefs are shaped by your emotions and vice versa. A person's ideas and emotions can talk to one another through the mind-body link.

The word "feeling" suggests a physical sense, even if your emotions are something you may only be aware of in your mind. Experiencing emotions is a physical event. There are physical sensations associated with every emotion you experience.

When you're feeling confident versus anxious, what goes through your mind? When you're apprehensive, you could start to feel that the end of the world is near. You may have negative thoughts about yourself, like that you are fragile or in danger. When you're feeling good about yourself, it's natural to assume those positive qualities extend to your mental fortitude.

Changing your physical stance can have a profound effect on your mood. Try to keep your head up and your shoulders back whenever you feel nervous or irritated. Your altered state of mind may come as a complete surprise to you.

As such, the mind-body connection is an integral part of the treatment of mental health and substance use problems. The mind-body link has beneficial effects on many aspects of health, including but not limited to sleep, diet, exercise, and general mobility.

When you're anxious, for instance, that feeling could start in your stomach. A heightened heart rate is possible. The instinct to shield yourself may cause you to adopt a more closed posture.

If you're feeling good about yourself, you might even straighten up and carry yourself with pride. You are able to regulate your breathing and heart rate. Maybe you'll feel confident and at peace. As your emotions change, so will your thinking.

Because the body exerts an impact over the mind and vice versa, understanding the mind-body link is crucial to maintaining mental health and overcoming addiction.

The mind-body link is important, and it is recommended that mental health and substance misuse treatment programs incorporate mind-body exercises. You can improve both your physical and mental health at the same time.

It is possible to include mind-body ideas into treatment for mental health and addiction. You'll have more resources for healing at your disposal thanks to these vital mind-body therapies.

THE MIND BODY RELATIONSHIP WHAT IS IT AND WHY SHOULD I CARE

The term "mind-body connection" refers to the relationship between a person's mental and physical well-being.

Although it has been known for some time that our feelings have physical consequences, only recently have we started to comprehend the role that our feelings play in our overall health and lifespan.

Holistic medicine, a healthcare philosophy that aims to treat the whole person rather than just the symptoms, places a strong emphasis on the mind-body relationship. As the need for healing on all levels (mental, physical, and spiritual) becomes more apparent, medical professionals are increasingly emphasizing holistic approaches to treatment.

FACILITATING A BETTER BRAIN BODY CONNECTION

It makes sense that this is commonly referred to as the "mind-body link," since it is essential for the proper operation of both the body and the mind. We've compiled a list of 21 effective actions that could help you reestablish and fortify this incredibly advantageous equilibrium.

THE BENEFITS OF MEDITATION CANNOT BE OVERSTATED

The mind and body can be brought closer together via the practice of meditation. By the end of the session, your body will feel rested and your mind will be calm and alert. Through regular meditation practice, one can overcome emotional stress and enjoy a state of deep calm. There is evidence that practicing mindfulness for as little as 10 to 15 minutes a day might alleviate symptoms of stress, anxiety, and chronic pain.

LEARN TO TAKE DEEP BREATHS

Restoring mental and physical equilibrium by concentration on the breath is a simple yet effective technique. By taking a few slow, deep breaths, you can potentially boost your focus on the here and now, reduce your heart rate and blood pressure, and lessen the effects of the "fight or flight" stress reaction. Just close your eyes, inhale deeply enough to fill your diaphragm, then exhale slowly a few more times. You will be calmer and more attuned to your environment, but also more prepared to respond to any potential threats.

PRESERVE A BALANCED DIET

If you want to maintain good mental and physical health, you need to take care of your body from the inside out, and that includes eating right. It is important to eat nutritious food and to eat it in a mindful manner. Dietitians advise eating foods that are fresh, freshly prepared, and varied in color, and avoiding foods that are canned, frozen, microwaved, or overly processed, as well as including all six basic flavors (sweet, salty, sour, pungent, bitter, and astringent) in each meal.

AVOID DEHYDRATION BY MAINTAINING AN ADEQUATE FLUID INTAKE

Depending on our weight, water might make up as much as 60% of our bodies. Each and every one of your body's cells, tissues, and organs can't do their jobs without being adequately hydrated. Headaches, weariness, and other symptoms of dehydration have been seen in scientific studies. Therefore, it is essential to drink water regularly no matter how busy we are, and this holds true even while we are on the go.

GET PLENTY OF REST

To maintain health and vigor, a good night's sleep is crucial. Inadequate sleep has been linked to mood and energy swings, a weakened immune system, and a host of other negative health outcomes. An adult need eight hours of sleep per night, and falling asleep fast without the aid of drugs or alcohol is essential if you want to get the most out of those hours. You know you got quality sleep when you wake up feeling refreshed, revitalized, and full of life.

TIME SPENT IN NATURE IS TIME WELL SPENT

It has been shown that at least 120 minutes a week spent outside has positive effects on one's mental and physical health. Nature therapy is a great way to cleanse your head and relax your senses. Simply put, being outside makes you feel more in one with the real world. Getting some outdoor air is good for your health and your longevity no matter what the weather is like.

GET SOME SORT OF REGULAR WORKOUT

Exercising on a regular basis has enormous positive effects on your body and mind. Physical activity not only maintains a healthy, strong, and youthful body, but also improves the brain's cognitive capabilities and fosters a state of positive emotion. Cardiovascular activity, strength training, and stretching are the three cornerstones of a well-rounded fitness routine. If you want to increase your physical and mental energy, try exercising for at least 20 to 30 minutes every day.

DO SOME YOGA

Asanas (physical postures) and pranayama (breathing techniques) are the foundation of yoga, an age-old and supreme mind-body practice. Its peaceful, relaxing, and tranquil features help your mind reconnect with the physical sensations in your body as you lengthen and strengthen your muscles, improve your balance, and expand your range of motion.

REFRESH YOURSELF WITH SOME PHYSICAL ACTIVITY DURING BREAKS

Taking breaks that involve physical activity are another great method to get out of your head and back into your body. Try to get up and move around every hour to help keep your body from feeling sluggish. Removing yourself from a stressful situation can help your brain come up with a more workable answer.

DITCH THE BAD FEELINGS

Unresolved feelings of hurt, disappointment, or rage may be extremely harmful to the mind and body, and they may be holding you back from reaching your full potential without your even recognizing it. Ask yourself what you did in the past that no longer serves you emotionally or mentally. Think about how much better your life will be when you've dealt with them, and then tell yourself that you're really doing it this time.

SEIZE THE DAY

Hone your ability to feel good by embracing positive states of mind such as contentment, pleasure, love, and gratitude. If you want to have more time for spontaneity and enjoyment in the here and now, it's a good idea to regularly assess your work, home, social, and online activities to see what may be cut or shortened.

LAUGH YOUR HEARTS OUT

Research has shown that laughter can have positive effects on health by decreasing the body's generation of stress hormones and increasing the immune system's resistance. Laughter instantly improves our mood by stimulating our heart, lungs, and muscles. Try to find something humorous to watch once a day so you can let loose with a good belly laugh.

SHOW GRATITUDE

Practicing gratitude is like doing yoga for your brain. Aside from making you happier and less depressed, it also stimulates your brain to release endorphins, which have a plethora of beneficial effects on your body and mind. If you want to feel more fulfilled in life, less materialistic, and more spiritually connected, try practicing the art of gratitude.

PRESERVE A DIARY

One of the best ways to deal with the stresses of daily life is to keep a journal. Writing things down helps you get them out of your head and reduces anxiety so you can tackle the matter more rationally. Keeping a gratitude notebook is another common activity. Taking the time to reflect on the blessings in your life and record them on paper can have a profoundly good effect on your mental and emotional health.

CURB YOUR SCREEN TIME

Technology such as smartphones, social media, and television can be huge time wasters and cause a sense of alienation very immediately. To be more present and to live a richer and more involved life, it is crucial to learn to power off the devices. Start with a daily digital detox of 20–30 minutes and work your way up to an afternoon or even a weekend. Getting off electronics at least an hour before bedtime has been shown to improve sleep quality.

ENGAGE IN HEARTWARMING INTERACTIONS

Our emotional and physical health are profoundly influenced by the quality of the relationships we maintain. Having friends and family by your side helps alleviate feelings of isolation, provides sound counsel in times of crisis, and encourages you to work through challenging times. Spending time with them can be a welcome diversion from your concerns.

MAKE SURE YOU'RE SITTING OR STANDING UPRIGHT CORRECTLY

It's been scientifically shown that our body postures affect our emotions, not merely reflect them. Putting on an air of confidence can be as simple as standing up straight and holding your head high. It's important to pay attention to someone's facial expressions as well, since the brain interprets those as emotional cues. Smiling is a technique that, when practiced, can lead to an increase in positive emotions.

APPRECIATE THE GIFTS OF YOUR SENSES

The demands of daily life might cause us to neglect our innate abilities to perceive the world around us through our senses of sight, sound, taste, and touch. It doesn't take much work, though, to interact with them and return your focus to your physical self. If you find yourself longing for these emotions in the midst of your workday, keeping a bottle of essential oil on your desk or draping a comfy blanket over your chair may assist. Even on your busiest days, take a few minutes to sit down and savor your meal. Consider getting a massage when you get home from work to unwind, increase your blood flow, and calm down.

ENJOY SOME TUNES

Music is a wonderful and pleasurable medium for reacquainting yourself with your bodily senses. Singing or dancing to your favorite tune might help release negative feelings that have been weighing you down. You may take charge of your mood, improve your disposition, and gain confidence and motivation by listening to music that mirrors the energy you wish to experience.

GET SERIOUS ABOUT A CREATIVE PURSUIT

You can enter a contemplative state of mind by engaging in artistic pursuits like painting, sculpting, playing an instrument, or even cooking. Such pursuits have been shown to alleviate tension and anxiety, as well as aid in the resolution of both internal and external disputes. Learning and attempting new things is like giving your brain a workout; it increases your enthusiasm for life and your sense of pride in yourself.

THE NEUROCHEMICAL BASIS OF CONSCIOUSNESS

While there is much about the mind-body link that remains unknown, researchers are beginning to uncover how this relationship actually works. According to Dr. Jennifer Weinberg, MD, MPH, MBE, a specialist in preventive and lifestyle health, the brain is the "hardware" that gives us access to the range of mental states that we refer to as "mind."

Hormones and neurotransmitters are just two examples of chemical and physical messengers that facilitate communication. In fact, scientists have mapped the neurological pathways that send signals from the brain to the adrenal medulla during times of stress. These results shed light on how emotional states like stress and despair might affect bodily processes.

PHYSICAL CONDITION AND STRESS

Stressful emotions have been shown to lower immunity by influencing how the body's blood cells work. Anxiety dampens the immune system's ability to fight off infections and tumors, according to one study. People's immune systems become less responsive to immunizations and their wounds take longer to heal when they're under stress. In addition, CBT and other forms of talk therapy have been shown to improve cell function and, by extension, the immune system's capacity to fight off illness.

The effect of the mind-body link on a group of people who had previously survived breast cancer was the subject of a groundbreaking study. Some of the people in the study were able to reduce their stress levels by engaging in mindfulness meditation or going to a support group. Comparatively, those who did nothing served as the control group.

The protein complexes at the ends of chromosomes (telomeres) were found to be much longer in the meditation and support group groups compared to the control group. Disease is linked to shortened telomeres, while longer telomeres offer protection from illness.

THE RELATIONSHIP BETWEEN DIET AND MENTAL AND PHYSICAL HEALTH

The mind-body link is profoundly influenced by one's dietary habits.

What you put into your body has an immediate and direct effect on your state of mind. The destructive effects of drug misuse are something you can consider. Substance abuse can damage both the mind and the body. You can speed up the recovery process by eating well and staying sober.

When you're trying to recover from an addiction, a nutritious diet can help you heal both physically and mentally while avoiding relapse.

You'll have more energy and a better mood after eating something that's good for your brain and body. Consider how you'd feel after consuming a lot of sugar. You could have a high at first, followed by a low afterwards.

Eating junk food can make you feel terrible, but not as dreadful as you would feel after eating a decent meal. When overcoming mental health or addiction, proper nutrition can provide the vitality, energy, and minerals your body needs to heal.

The foods we eat have a direct effect on our brain chemistry and overall well-being. The food we eat can help us avoid or even overcome issues with our mental health. The SMILES Trial and other studies shown that the food we eat can affect how we feel. Some nutrients, in particular, have been related to noticeable improvements in psychological health.

The mind-body link is also reflected in the two-way dialogue between the brain and the digestive system. One of the main hormones in controlling mood and emotion is serotonin, and around 95% of it is created in the digestive tract. This enteric (intestinal-related) nervous system, sometimes known as the "second brain" or the "belly brain," comprises of about 100 million neurons sheaths of neurons buried in the walls of the gut. More importantly, the digestive system is the primary conduit for information transfer to the cerebral cortex.

Decreased rates of anxiety and depression have been linked to a more diversified and healthy microbiome, according to the study's authors. Furthermore, evidence from research in both animals and humans shows that introducing beneficial bacteria into the stomach can drastically influence mood and emotional regulation.

Chapter 2

AGGRESSIVE MENTAL ATTITUDES

But having a positive mental attitude involves more than just not giving up. True power of mind comes from a mix of awareness, attention and resiliency. A positive frame of mind is what keeps you intent on your goals rather than dwelling on setbacks. What you need to learn is that setbacks are temporary and need not derail your progress toward achievement. It prevents you from making choices that would lead to harming yourself.

How, therefore, can you train your mind so that it can compete with that of the greatest athletes on the planet? You pick up and begin using the same routines they do. To help you cultivate a similar winning mindset, we've compiled ten habits of really successful people.

THEY MAKE ADVANTAGE OF THE POTENTIAL OF THOUGHT

At the recent Human Gathering conference in Los Angeles, I had the pleasure of meeting Randy Jackson, the former host of American Idol and a prominent business leader in the music industry. Artists like David Bowie and Madonna, he said, had a mentality that led to an unquenchable faith in their own future achievement. Even before they achieved fame and fortune, they carried themselves as if it were inevitable.

This is a perfect illustration of the way that successful people use the potential of intention to form underlying convictions about the outcomes they seek. Once they're satisfied, they materialize it. You can learn to channel this energy by meditating on the following collection of mantras, which have been shown to be effective in creating a winning mentality.

THEY SCHEDULE IN CONTEMPLATION TIME

While successful people do have full schedules, they don't spend all their time with their heads down grinding away. Additionally, they recognize the value of thinking things out and contemplation. They regularly evaluate their work and give their thoughts the breathing room they need to come up with novel concepts or seize unexpected possibilities.

THEY FIGURE OUT HOW TO COMBAT THEIR OWN DEPRESSING IDEAS

The highest achievers are those who recognize the destructive patterns of thought that plague the majority of people and have developed effective strategies for overcoming them. Instead of trying to push unpleasant thoughts out of their heads, they recognize that they are just that—thoughts. They avoid being emotionally invested, which allows them to view familiar situations from fresh perspectives. The final step is to substitute a more beneficial thinking for the negative one.

THEY DISREGARD THEIR DETRACTORS

There will always be naysayers when you go for the gusto. No one who wants to succeed lets negativity or the opinions of others dampen their aspirations or sense of self-worth.

THEY SIT IN QUIET CONTEMPLATION

As a form of self-awareness, meditation helps you quiet your mind and tune in to your internal experiences. Although there are many different ways to meditate and many different tools available, the end result is the same: a deeper understanding of who you are and a reduced stress and anxiety baseline. Successful people realize that silence is the best way to clear their minds of tension and distractions and allow creative ideas to flow freely in the desired direction.

IN THIS CONTEXT THEY COLLABORATE WITH TRAINERS

Those at the top of their game often work with coaches to help them maintain a laser-like concentration, hold them accountable, and polish their skills. They recognize that working with a coach is essential to developing their skills and potential.

CONTINUALLY EXPANDING THEIR KNOWLEDGE

Amazing achievers tend to share a passion

for reading and education. People who go far in life tend to devour books. They understand that the foundation of a growth mentality is a thirst for knowledge. If you're an entrepreneur, check out this reading list.

THEIR AIMS ARE CRYSTALLIZED

Those that succeed in life are able to articulate their desires. They set attainable, detailed objectives and commit them to paper. Putting thoughts to paper gives them more weight and substance. Furthermore, many prosperous people make use of vision boards as a means of constantly reminding themselves of their goals.

THEY KEEP ACTIVE BY WORKING OUT

Although we are all aware of the health benefits associated with physical activity, we rarely make it a top priority. Extremely successful people understand the link between mental and physical fitness and career advancement. The mental and physical challenges you'll face on your route to greatness will be easier to bear if you're in good shape.

THE TWO OF THEM HAD A GOOD TIME AND LAUGH

Laughter is a great way to let go of tension and negative emotions because it triggers the release of endorphins, the brain's "feel good" hormone. Positive emotions and increased output are common among those who laugh frequently. Put some humor into your day, even if it's just a five minute.

The ups and downs of starting and running your own business are far more manageable if you have a solid mental foundation. When your faculties are low from exhaustion, fear, or panic, you are more likely to make poor choices. Incorporate these practices into your life to strengthen your mind and propel you forward in your pursuit of happiness and success.

ALTER YOUR FRAME OF THOUGHT

Your frame of mind can have a huge impact on how you deal with any given scenario and the results you achieve. Your coaching, profession, business, and general happiness can all benefit greatly from adjusting your frame of thinking. A negative frame of mind is easy to adopt and difficult to abandon. Once you're not in the appropriate frame of mind, you'll notice that things don't appear to go your way. This is because you're focusing on the negatives rather than the positives.

The best educational opportunities can alter our perceptions of who we are, how we relate to others, and what our place is in the world. Learning, the acquisition of expertise, social interactions, personal growth, and professional and personal accomplishments are only few of the spheres of life that can be influenced by one's mindset. Therefore, whether your goal is to succeed in the fitness business, advance in your work, or accomplish something else entirely, the key is to develop a more positive mental attitude. Well, how exactly do you accomplish that? Well, read on for some terrific advice on how to adjust your frame of mind:

GROW FROM YOUR ERRORS

Mistakes are inevitable; that's just how life is. What separates the successful from the unsuccessful is that the former learn from their blunders while the latter allow them to drag them up. Take the negative experiences you've had and turn them into learning opportunities. Do not look at this setback as a failure, but rather as an opportunity to develop and improve. It didn't work out this time, but you've learned from your mistakes and will tackle the problem differently next time.

FOCUS ON THE LITTLE THINGS

It's easy to set unrealistic goals for oneself and judge one's progress in the fitness sector when one is just starting out. It's easy to lose sight of your progress toward success if you keep focusing on the fact that you haven't yet accomplished everything you set out to do. Make an effort to set frequent, minor goals, and reward yourself when you reach them.

EXERT SOME PLIABILITY

To keep a positive frame of mind, it's important to be able to adapt when things aren't going as planned. As the saying goes, "life doesn't always go the way you intend, but that's just a lesson you can learn from." By keeping an open mind and being adaptable to life's inevitable twists and turns as well as the inevitable setbacks, you can avoid feeling defeated and instead find the strength to persevere. Always keep in mind that tomorrow is a fresh start, so if today didn't go as planned, make tomorrow your day!

GAIN MOTIVATION

Aspirational thinking is the result of being inspired. Engage in a daily ritual that serves to renew your spirit. It might be anything from a meeting with like-minded people to viewing a motivational lecture online. The key is to actively seek it out, because inspiration is everywhere.

TAKE A FEW MOMENTS FOR YOURSELF TO RELAX AND REFLECT

Every day, give yourself a few minutes to relax and recharge by spending time alone. Some people like to be the first ones out of bed in the morning, while others prefer the peace and quiet of the evening hours. Take a few minutes to yourself whenever you can, even if you're extremely busy, and go to a peaceful place. The simple act of taking five or ten minutes for yourself multiple times a day can do wonders for your mental health, especially if you're starting to feel frustrated, overwhelmed, sad, or furious.

When you have some alone time, try some deep breathing exercises while thinking about anything or somewhere that calms and soothes you. If you find yourself thinking something negative, just push it out of your mind and replace it with something positive. In the end, you'll have a sense of peace and relaxation that will help you tackle the challenges ahead with a more optimistic outlook.

HONOR WHAT YOU HAVE BY SHOWING GRATITUDE

Focusing on the positive aspects of your life can be challenging if you're dealing with stress at work, school, or at home. When things don't go as planned or you feel misunderstood and ignored, it's tempting to wallow in self-pity and focus on what you don't have. You might even start wondering why you have to go through this, but it won't change anything.

If you find yourself dwelling on the negative, try redirecting your attention to the many wonderful aspects of your life. If you're healthy, have a supportive network of friends and family, live in a comfortable house, and have a rewarding career, you have plenty to be thankful for. You could even benefit from keeping a tiny notepad on you at all times to jot down your thoughts of gratitude as they come to you. There's a good chance that, over time, you'll compile a lengthy list that will serve to put things in perspective and immediately lift your mood.

Every day, jot down three things for which you are thankful. You won't have to devote a lot of time to this straightforward thankfulness activity. It's a simple approach to get into a routine of daily gratitude, which is appreciated by many.

TAKE PART IN A REWARDING DIALOGUE

Ever notice how animated you become when discussing topics that truly fascinate you? As enthusiasm takes hold, you feel a rush of joy and your heart rate increases somewhat. It's a great emotion that makes you believe you can achieve any goal you set for yourself.

That's why changing one's mood for the better may be as simple as striking up a conversation with someone you know, whether they're a family member, coworker, or even a nice stranger. Whenever you engage in conversation about topics that bring you joy, you can't help but feel better. Your outlook on life improves, and as a result, so does your general disposition.

PUT ON A HAPPY FACE AND HELP SOMEONE ELSE OUT

A cheerful disposition can lift the spirits of others around you as well as your own. When you smile, you immediately improve your mood and the mood of those around you. The minor things that may typically ruin your day become less noticeable. Give to others if you can't seem to make yourself happy. This simple act of kindness, such as holding a door open for someone, never fails to put a smile on your face.

Smiling is contagious and can help you meet new and fascinating individuals because people appreciate being around those who are positive and approachable. It's possible that this will lead to a whole new world of incredible possibilities and uplifting adventures. So, when you feel yourself spiraling into despair, stop, breathe deeply, force a grin across your face, and go out of your way to do something kind for someone else. Eventually, you'll feel the good vibes emanating from every direction.

TAKE CARE WITH YOUR WORD CHOICE

A person's frame of mind can be inferred not only from the way they think, but also from the words they choose to use. How often do you tell yourself that you can't accomplish anything or that the day is just doomed to be bad? Dispositive energy is generated by negative speech. The more you use them, the more bad luck you attract. If you tell yourself you're going to have a bad day, you're more likely to really experience a poor day.

To attract positive energy and move you closer to your goals, replace negative language with more upbeat expressions. Tell yourself that today is going to be great and that you are up to whatever challenges you may face. You may boost your confidence, vitality, and enthusiasm for life by surrounding yourself with uplifting words.

MAINTAIN A NEUTRAL PERSPECTIVE

If you believe you have limited potential, you will never reach your full potential. You're limiting your potential by refusing to consider new options. It's understandable if you start to question the value of your efforts when faced with such limited potential outcomes. Depression and anxiety are inevitable outcomes.

The good news is that you can immediately change your outlook by adopting a more open stance. It encourages you to believe in yourself and pursue lofty goals so that you can develop intellectually and personally. You'll have the drive to make the adjustments that will enhance every facet of your life.

Use one or more of the above strategies to strengthen your frame of mind when dealing with adversity and toxic environments that foster negative thinking. You can live a happier, more productive life by adopting a positive outlook on life and working hard to realize your full potential in all that you do.

If you want to take charge of your life, you need to take charge of your thoughts. Instead of passively letting life pass you by, you can actively decide how you want to live and what you want to accomplish. Whenever you feel a cloud of pessimism settling over your mind, stop what you're doing and devote a few minutes to thinking positively instead. It will boost your confidence and encourage you to keep moving forward.

Chapter 3

CONSIDER YOUR MENTAL AND PHYSICAL WELL BEING

To be physically healthy is to possess a physique that is robust, able, and disease-free. Having a mind that is robust, capable, and disease-free is what we mean when we talk about mental health.

OPTIMISM AND THE HEALING ARTS

The mind-body connection is far more powerful than the average person realizes; our emotions are directly tied to how we see the world around us. Even as we try to imagine what might happen in the future, our bodies are already reacting to the thought.

Think about what you'll do if someone cuts you off and almost causes an accident the next time it happens. Even if your meeting only lasts a fraction of a second, your body has began to prepare for the worst case scenario by creating a surge of adrenaline. One such bodily reaction is the rush of adrenaline. From changes in blood pressure and heart rate to shifts in brain chemistry, the human mind may bring about these and other physiological responses merely by thinking about it. Acutely, these changes might not be dangerous to your health, but they could have dire consequences later on.

Every once in a while, we look back on a decision and wonder how we came to make it. It might be as simple as making the choice to eat a cheeseburger when you had planned on eating healthier. The consequences of one's actions magnify when the stakes are higher, as when one flirts with a married coworker. In order to learn more about the human brain and how it works...

Many of our past actions and choices raise doubts when seen in retrospect. The smallest of decisions, like opting for a cheeseburger when you promised yourself you'd eat healthier, can have the biggest impact. For example, flirting with a married coworker can have serious consequences.

In order to fully understand how our thoughts affect our daily lives, one must first recognize the intricate web of connections that makes up our society. A more detailed breakdown of these variables includes the following.

THOUGHTS

We have thoughts because the brain receives and processes information. The mind acts as the checkpoint for the computer's processing mechanism. We focus on the information it deems most crucial. There is a risk that these notions will harden into firm convictions, which will in turn mold our feelings.

Just consider the cheeseburger. Maybe you were thinking, "I'm starving" or "I've had such a rough day, I deserve a treat."

FEELINGS

A person's feelings are the end outcome of their own thoughts and deeds. They show how invested we are in a given activity. Humans are the source of them because of the wealth of experience and many perspectives we bring to the table.

Here's where things may get sticky: even a statement as simple as "I am hungry" might be loaded with emotional connotations that have little to do with actual hunger. It's easy to associate the words "I'm hungry" with a wide range of negative emotions, from stress at work to anger after an argument to despair after hearing bad news.

BEHAVIORS

The mental and emotional conditions of an individual are reflected in their conduct. Our minds convince us that doing some action is in our best interest whenever we do it in reaction to something.

As a result, if you're hungry and also feeling sad, stressed out, etc., you might determine that eating a cheeseburger is the best solution.

There is a clear and strong connection between these three unique categories.

When we really give mind to how powerful our thoughts are, we see how they permeate every facet of our lives. They cause us to feel and act in certain ways. Everything from our mood to our actions is influenced by our mental pictures of the situation.

If you often find yourself regretting how you responded, maintaining a journal can help. What's your internal monologue like? How do you feel about yourself, the other people involved, and the situation as a whole.

HOW TO CHANGE YOUR MINDSET AND BECOME MORE POSITIVE

Are you constantly thinking negatively? You aren't helping yourself if your inner monologue is often critical of others and, by extension, yourself. Psychologist Scott Bea, PsyD., discusses the prevalence of pessimistic thought patterns and offers advice for shifting to a more optimistic worldview.

CAN YOU NAME ANY OF THE ISSUES THAT A NEGATIVE OUTLOOK CAUSES

Feeling down about life, oneself, and one's future is a direct result of dwelling on the negative. It's a factor that makes you feel bad about yourself. It makes you feel helpless and useless.

Experts in psychology have found a connection between pessimistic thoughts and mental health issues like depression, anxiety, and (OCD). The vast majority of people struggle with it, including those who are naturally optimistic.

This is because of the inherent structure of human brains. The amygdala and the rest of the limbic system in our brain are set up to detect danger and take appropriate action to ensure our survival. The savannah could have been picturesque on a sunny day in prehistoric times, but we were conditioned to recognize the threat posed by a nearby predator.

The same regions of the brain are now engaged even when actual danger is low. Nowadays, we have to deal with more mental dangers, such as worries about money, relationships, and professional advancement. They have the potential to increase our heart rates. So much so that just thinking about going into the office on Monday causes us to freak out on a Sunday

The answer is yes, it is possible to develop a habit of thinking negatively.

Absolutely. Through repetition, we learn to worry more effectively. Ritualized reassurance is what keeps worry at bay. To calm ourselves, we imagine the worst-case scenarios and then plan for how to get through them.

However, confidence is like coffee in that its effects wear off quickly. If you're using coffee to stay awake, know that the more you drink, the more tired you'll eventually feel. People who say things like "The older I get, the more I worry," have likely been practicing those words.

Even if we try to predict every possible outcome of the story, it will only end in one manner. There is a 94% chance that our worst fears will never come true. Often, the things that actually occur are completely unexpected.

The media constantly injects us with pessimism by focusing almost exclusively on tragic stories. That we are more interested in wrongdoing than in right doing is something they have observed.

IS IT EVEN FEASIBLE TO ALTER ONE'S MENTAL PROCESSES

As opposed to altering your cognitive processes, you should shift your perspective on and response to your thoughts instead. About 50,000 random thoughts, images, and ideas pop into our heads every day. These thoughts, whether pleasant or bad, force themselves into our consciousness. Negative statements are more likely to linger in our minds.

Learning to observe your ideas rather than participating in them is something I would advise. Mindfulness is a technique that can help you stop thinking for a while.

For instance

Take five to ten seconds to focus on your breathing or your footfall.

Take note of everything that distracts you from focusing on them.

Then, bring your attention back to your breath or your steps.

If you find yourself dwelling on something terrible, remind yourself to bring your attention back to the here and now. Describe what your senses are revealing to you at the moment.

Practicing mindfulness also helps us hardwire a moral compass. What's working in the here and now can be systematically noted. In every individual we meet, there is a positive trait we may observe. Appropriateness can be better seen when accompanied by words of praise.

A notebook of thanksgiving can help us focus on the positive outcomes. It's best to do this just before bed for maximum effect.

CAN YOU PHYSICALLY ALTER YOUR BRAIN BY THINKING POSITIVELY

We now know that a person's brain chemistry may be altered through deliberate effort to alter their habits. Because of how deeply ingrained habits are in the brain, replacing them with better ones is a challenge.

The opposite is true with new habits, which tend to become embedded and almost unconscious after repeated use. At first, we could fight against a fitness routine, but eventually, it just becomes second nature. We can apply this same principle to our relationship with our thoughts by attempting to establish new routines.

For this reason, mindfulness is increasingly being employed in the treatment of conditions such as social anxiety, obsessive-compulsive disorder, and depression. Mindfulness teaches us to be content with our circumstances rather than constantly searching for ways to improve them.

WHAT CHANGES AS YOU ADOPT A MORE OPTIMISTIC OUTLOOK

How you think about life changes how you feel about it. Self-love and confidence are cultivated through optimistic thought.

Perhaps you've been blessed with an ability that can improve the lives of those around you. The effect of praise on others is profound. In other words, it makes people happy. To put it simply, it improves our health, our productivity, and the state of the globe.

Increasing your level of optimism can help you see things in a new light, which may lead to a more effective method of doing your job. As a lawyer, for instance, you may find that taking a more supportive stance benefits your clients.

Increasing our capacity for positive can even change our actions, improving our well being and the results we see in our life.

HOW TO TAKE CHARGE OF YOUR MIND AND STOP ALLOWING IT TO CONTROL YOU

One's own mind is capable of great good or great harm, depending on how it is employed. If you can manage your thoughts, you can shape your behavior.

What you think, and hence how you see the world, is influenced by what you think about. And this is why what you see is what you get:

Somewhere about 70,000 thoughts every day is the norm, so I've been told. If they are unmotivated, abusive to themselves, and a drain on resources, that's a lot of people.

You're free to let your mind wander, but why bother? To what extent have you felt the need to reclaim control of your own mind and ideas? Would you agree that you need to start making decisions now?

Determine to be the one who is intentionally, actively thinking these words. Become a person whose mind is their own master by learning to regulate and direct their own ideas.

When you alter the way you think, you not only alter the way you feel, but you also remove the causes of your negative emotions. Both of these results will provide you more mental tranquility.

Several random notions have recently entered my mind, and they are neither my choice nor a result of my retraining. Now that I have learned to control my thoughts, my mind is at peace. And so can yours!

The first step toward regaining mental

control is realizing that multiple uninvited "squatters" have set up shop in your brain.

To take control and kick them out, you need to first understand who they are and what drives them.

LEARNING TO THINK AND TALK POSITIVELY

Think positively without denying the reality of unpleasant circumstances. Simply said, positive thinking entails taking a brighter and more fruitful tack while dealing with challenges. You anticipate the best outcomes rather than the worst ones.

Self-talk is frequently the first step toward positive thinking. The constant chatter of your own mind is known as self-talk. Both good and negative thoughts can arise automatically. You use rational thought in some of your internal dialogue. It's also possible that your internal dialogue is influenced by false beliefs you hold about yourself or the world around you owing to a lack of knowledge or the application of unrealistic assumptions.

If you tend to dwell on the negative, you are more likely to have a gloomy attitude on life. You are an optimist, or someone who uses positive thinking, if you tend to think positively most of the time.

THE FAVORABLE EFFECTS OF OPTIMISM ON HEALTH

The benefits of optimism and a positive outlook on health are still being investigated. Among the possible health benefits of maintaining an optimistic outlook are Lengthened longevity

Reduced occurrences of depression

Minimized Anguish and Pain

Improved health and immunity

Improvements in both mental and

physical health

Improvements in heart health and a lower chance of dying from cardiovascular causes and stroke

The possibility of dying from cancer is lowered.

fewer deaths from respiratory diseases Lessening of the likelihood of contracting and dying from infections superior ability to deal with adversity and pressure It is not known why optimistic thinkers reap these health benefits. It has been hypothesized that a more optimistic mindset mitigates the negative physiological impacts of stress.

It has also been hypothesized that persons who are naturally upbeat and optimistic tend to lead healthier lives overall. Recognizing unfavorable mental processes Worried that you may be talking negatively to yourself but unsure of the source. Examples of common forms of negative self-talk include.

FILTERING

As a result of this, you only see the negative features of a situation and ignore the favorable ones. Perhaps you have a successful day in the office. You finished everything ahead of schedule, and your efficiency and attention to detail earned you praise. At home that night, all you can think about is how you're going to get even more done, and you let the praises slip your mind.

Personalizing. It's human nature to feel responsible for one's own misfortune when it occurs. If, for instance, you learn that a night out with friends has been postponed, you might conclude that your pals decided to ditch the outing because they no longer wish to spend time with you.

Catastrophizing. Your mind immediately jumps to the worst case scenario, even though you have no reason to believe it is actually possible. Having your drive-through coffee order botched makes you feel like the rest of your day is doomed to failure.

BLAMING

You make an attempt to shift blame away from yourself and onto another party. You try to avoid taking accountability for how you actually feel.

A recommendation that you "should" take action. You beat yourself up mentally for failing to accomplish the things you know you should.

Magnifying. You tend to overreact to relatively insignificant situations.

Perfectionism. Failure is inevitable if you hold yourself to standards that are impossible to meet.

POLARIZING

You only ever see things in black and white. In this case, neither side is budging.

Keeping a bright outlook Altering your default mode of thinking from pessimistic to optimistic is something you can train yourself to do. Even though it's easy to accomplish, it will require some effort on your part to form this new habit. Here are a few suggestions for adopting a more upbeat and optimistic mindset and style of life.

FIND WHAT NEEDS TO BE ALTERED

Whether it's job, your daily commute, life changes, or a relationship, pinpointing the specific situations in which you tend to think negatively is the first step toward adopting a more positive outlook and thinking style. Start by picking one facet of your life that you want to approach more optimistically. You can better cope with stress by replacing negative thoughts with more optimistic ones.

Get your head on straight. You should take a moment to assess your mental state at regular intervals during the day. If you discover that you are dwelling on unpleasant things, it may help to reframe such thoughts.

Have a good sense of humor. Laugh or smile at yourself, even if you're going through a tough period. Seek out the funny in common occurrences. Having a good sense of humor helps reduce anxiety.

ADOPT A BALANCED HEALTHY ROUTINE

Aim for 30-minute workouts five days a week. You can do this in 5- or 10-minute intervals spread out throughout the day. Exercising has been shown to improve mood and alleviate stress. Take care of your body and mind by eating right. The importance of getting enough sleep cannot be overstated. As well as find effective methods of dealing with stress.

Put yourself in an environment full of upbeat people. It's important to surround yourself with upbeat, encouraging people who will encourage you and provide constructive criticism. If you're around a lot of negative people, you could start to feel overwhelmed and start to doubt your own ability to deal with stress in a healthy way.

BE ENCOURAGING TO YOURSELF

First, don't talk to yourself in a way that you wouldn't talk to a close friend or loved one. Treat yourself with kindness and support. If a negative thought occurs to you, give it a sober assessment and counter it with positive self-affirmations. Consider the many blessings you now enjoy.

Chapter 4

IN TERMS OF BOTH YOUR MENTAL AND PHYSICAL HEALTH

We've covered how stress can wreak havoc on your health, but what about the other way around?

Our mental and physical wellness are intrinsically connected. Our resistance to chronic diseases and our propensity to make good decisions are both diminished by poor mental and physical health. When our mental health declines, our physical health follows behind.

Keep in mind that stress is a known threat to your health. Excessive stress is associated with an increased vulnerability to clinical depression. A person's happiness plummets once they've been diagnosed with depression. Once this occurs, the individual's physical health deteriorates as well.

Although depression is classified as a mental illness, it can have physical consequences.

Some people with depression experience a wide range of symptoms, including those related to their sexuality, their weight, their digestion, their ability to remember things, their ability to form new memories, and much more.

THE CONNECTION BETWEEN PSYCHOLOGICAL AND PHYSIOLOGICAL WELLBEING

Mental health has very substantial and far-reaching effects on physical health, just as well-being does. When you're mentally healthy, you're more likely to take care of your body.

SOME EXAMPLES THAT PROVE MY POINT

Maintaining a healthy lifestyle, which includes

eating well, getting plenty of water and exercise, and getting enough sleep, can help avoid or lessen the severity of mental health problems like depression and anxiety.

People with mental health problems, such as sadness and anxiety, can get well with the aid of a healthy lifestyle.

You can't have good mental health without also taking care of your body.

METHODS FOR IMPROVING ONE'S HEALTH

Including some new practices into your routine is all it takes to improve your well-being.

MAKE FRIENDS WITH PEOPLE

The quality of our social connections has a direct impact on our happiness and mental health. For obvious reasons: people thrive in communities. We're social creatures that thrive when we're surrounded by other people. Evolutionarily speaking, it was crucial to our continued existence.

Although we no longer live in tribal communities, we still need to have meaningful relationships in order to thrive. One of the many ways in which meaningful connections benefit us is by encouraging us to lead healthier lives.

Even while meeting new people in the post-modern world can be challenging, there are still many opportunities to develop meaningful connections with others. In order to help you out, I have compiled a list of some possible alternatives.

Connect with someone special over a video call using FaceTime or Zoom.

Make sure you spend some quality time with your spouse, roommates, children, or anybody else you call home.

Get to know your neighbors better by hosting a get-together in a public space, such as a driveway or a front step, and strengthening your shaky social ties.

Let a friend know you're thinking about them by sending them a text.

Start a virtual book group! The steps are as follows.

Take your special someone on a walk outside, where the two of you can enjoy some alone time without worrying about being overheard.

EXERT YOURSELF PHYSICALLY

Did you know that working out can make you feel better all around, from helping you sleep to boosting your mood to alleviating stress and depression.

Several scientific studies have shown that moderate depression can be efficiently treated through physical activity to the same degree as with leading antidepressant medicines, but without the negative side effects.

Starting off slowly is a good way to gain the health advantages of exercise. The chance of developing depression is reduced by 26% for every hour per day spent running or walking, according to research from the Harvard T.H. Chan School of Public Health.

OBTAIN CUTTING EDGE TRAINING

Learning new things throughout your life isn't simply a good way to pass the time; it's also a great method to keep your health in check.

Learning has been shown to delay cognitive decline, boost confidence and self-esteem, foster a sense of purpose, facilitate social ties, and even delay the onset of old age.

In light of this, it's time to go out and expand your knowledge. Learn a new language with an app like Duolingo, enroll in a course at a nearby college, or use edX to audit a course from one of the world's best universities at no cost. It's beneficial to your health and a lot of fun.

HELPING OTHERS IS GIVING TO YOURSELF

It's wonderful to help others, but does it actually boost your health? In a word, yeah.

You can start making a difference in the world by serving those closest to you. Find a local food bank or shelter in need of donations, or investigate local organizations that promote topics you care about.

There are countless opportunities to do good in the world, so it's easy to pick a cause that truly resonates with you.

DON'T WORRY ABOUT THE FUTURE; FOCUS ON THE HERE AND NOW

The tension of dwelling in the past or the anticipation of the future is something most of us can attest to from personal experience. It's easy to get stuck in the guilt, resentment, and regret that come along with dwelling on the past.

It's easy to let worry and excitement about the future overwhelm us when we let ourselves get caught up in it. Therefore, it is not surprising that being able to focus on the here and now is a necessary condition for flourishing.

mindfulness as "the practice of paying careful attention to one's experience in the present moment, without judging or analyzing it."

Mindfulness entails paying more attention to the present moment rather than dwelling on the past or future. Mindfulness has been shown to have numerous positive effects on health and well-being when practiced regularly.

Having less stress

reduced levels of stress and melancholy

improved disposition and perspective

Extra attention is needed.

One of the many apps out there can help you become more attentive in your daily life. Breathing exercises, walking meditation, yoga, and other such disciplines can also serve to ground you in the present moment.

START USING IT

To be fully effective, happy, and fulfilled as individuals, lovers, employees, and parents, health and well-being are not merely "good to have."

However, in today's fast-paced and frequently frantic environment, it's simple to neglect one's health and wellbeing.

Fortunately, there are many things we can do to boost our mental and physical health and well-being on a daily basis. This begins with recognizing what makes for happiness and how to generate more of it.

Daily improvements in health and happiness are possible through practices including meditation, service to others, physical activity, intellectual stimulation, and social interaction.

IS IT NOT VITAL THAT ONE MAINTAINS BOTH MENTAL AND PHYSICAL HEALTH

In what ways does one's mental health impact their physical well-being? When considering one's health as a whole, both mental and physical well-being are crucial. To give just a few examples, depression has been linked to an uptick in the risk of a wide range of physical health issues, especially chronic ones like diabetes, heart disease, and stroke.

CAN YOU DEFINE MENTAL HEALTH

When we say "mental health," we're referring to our emotional, psychological, and social states. The way we think, feel, and act are all influenced. It also plays a role in determining our stress responses, interpersonal connections, and dietary preferences. 1 Maintaining a healthy mental state is crucial at any age, from early childhood through adulthood.

Poor mental health and mental illness are not the same, despite common conflation of the two phrases. Even though a person has no diagnosable mental disorder, they may nonetheless be in a state of mental distress. A person with a mental disease can have times of health and happiness just like everyone else.

IN WHAT WAYS DOES ONE'S MENTAL HEALTH IMPACT THEIR PHYSICAL WELL-BEING?

When considering one's health as a whole, both mental and physical well-being are crucial. To give just a few examples, depression has been linked to an uptick in the risk of a wide range of physical health issues, especially chronic ones like diabetes, heart disease, and stroke. Similarly, having multiple chronic health problems may make you more vulnerable to mental illness.

CAN ONE'S MENTAL HEALTH IMPROVE WITH AGE

It's true that a person's mental health can evolve throughout time, influenced by a variety of factors. Stress can affect mental health when it forces people to use more energy and patience than they have. Inadequate mental health can be the result of many different factors, including but not limited to: working long hours, caring for a relative, or financial difficulties.

THE PREVALENCE OF MENTAL DISORDERS

In the United States, mental diseases are frequently seen.

In the course of a lifetime, more than half of the population will receive a diagnosis of a mental ailment or illness.

In any given year, one-fifth of Americans will suffer from a mental health issue.

One in five children will experience severe mental illness at some point in their lives.

Major depressive disorder, schizophrenia, and other severe mental illnesses affect 1 in 25 Americans.

JUST WHAT DO YOU DO TO MAKE SURE YOU'RE ALWAYS IN GOOD MENTAL AND BODILY HEALTH

Taking care of one's mental and emotional wellness

time well spent with trusted associates, family, and pals.

Communicate your feelings frequently.

cut back on your alcoholic beverages.

Keeping away from drugs that are illegal is the best option.

Keep moving and eating healthily.

gain experience and push your limits by learning something new.

Have fun and take it easy.

IS THERE A CONNECTION BETWEEN MENTAL AND PHYSICAL HEALTH

Mental and physical well-being are intertwined in ways that are often overlooked because of the widespread belief that the two are unrelated. A healthy mind can help you feel better physically. Inversely, if your mental health isn't up to par, it might take a toll on your body.

Mental health's influence on physical well-being

There is a strong correlation between your mental and physical wellness. A positive mental attitude can be protective against illness and prolong life. In a recent study, researchers discovered that people who reported higher levels of psychological well-being had lower rates of cardiovascular disease.

Conversely, issues with one's mental health can have negative effects on one's physical health and on the choices one makes.

Illnesses that last a long time. Many persistent diseases have been connected to depression.

Diabetes, asthma, cancer, cardiovascular disease, and arthritis are all examples of such conditions.

HEART AND LUNG PROBLEMS HAVE ALSO BEEN ASSOCIATED WITH SCHIZOPHRENIA

Having a mental health disorder can compound the challenges of living with a chronic condition. Depressed people and those with other mental health issues have a higher mortality rate from cancer and cardiovascular disease.

TROUBLE FALLING ASLEEP OR STAYING ASLEEP

Mentally ill people are disproportionately represented among those with sleep disorders like insomnia and apnea. Insomnia makes it difficult to get to sleep or remain asleep. Frequent awakenings are a common symptom of sleep apnea, which is caused by disruptions in breathing during sleep.

Individuals with mental health issues are twice as likely to have trouble sleeping as the general population. Ten percent to eighteen percent of the population has trouble sleeping.

Sleep problems are a double-edged sword: they can both cause and exacerbate mental health issues such as sadness, anxiety, and bipolar disorder.

SMOKING

More often than the general population, persons with mental health issues also smoke. People with mental health issues are disproportionately represented in the ranks of heavy smokers.

In depressed people, levels of the neurotransmitter dopamine are decreased. Dopamine is a neurotransmitter that helps you experience happiness. Since the nicotine in cigarettes stimulates the release of dopamine, this habit has been proposed as a treatment for depressive disorders.

ADVANTAGES IN OBTAINING MEDICAL ATTENTION

Unfortunately, those struggling with mental illness are disproportionately denied quality medical care.

People with mental health issues may also have a more difficult time prioritizing their physical health. It can be challenging to seek treatment, adhere to medication schedules, and maintain healthy lifestyle habits when dealing with a mental health disorder.

CONDITIONS OF THE BODY THAT MAY HAVE AN IMPACT ON THE MIND

Your mental health is affected by your physical health as well. Mental health problems are a risk factor for those with physical health problems.

Psoriasis is a skin disease that causes inflamed red patches. Acute stress and depression go hand in hand with it.

Psoriasis sufferers often struggle with mental anguish, which has a multiplicative effect on their health and standard of living. Anxiety, social stigma, and feeling rejected are major contributors to both stress and depression.

Depression and anxiety are common reactions to life-changing events like receiving a cancer diagnosis or recovering from a heart attack. Nearly a third of persons with life-threatening illnesses have depressive symptoms include poor mood, sleep disturbances, and a lack of interest in formerly pleasurable activities.

Tips for Maintaining Your Emotional and Physical Wellness Taking care of your physical and mental health is important if you want to feel better all around.

SOME SUGGESTIONS FOR TAKING CARE OF YOUR BODY AND MIND ARE AS FOLLOWS

Exercise frequently. Exercise not only aids in physical fitness, but it can also lift your spirits. The positive effects of a daily 10-minute walk include increased mental and physical energy and a better disposition.

Maintain a healthy diet. Physical and mental health can both benefit from a diet rich in fruits and vegetables and low in processed carbohydrates and fats. You may want to consult a registered dietitian for assistance in developing a diet program tailored to your specific requirements.

Just say no to drugs and booze. While alcohol and tobacco may temporarily improve your mood, in the long run they are harmful to your body and mind.

Be sure to get enough rest. 7–9 hours of sleep is ideal for people. If you need to feel more awake during the day, a 30-minute snooze may help.

Tend to your stress with some deep breathing exercises. If you're feeling stressed, try meditating, taking some deep breaths, and concentrating on one topic at a time.

Hone your thinking skills. Think about the good things that have happened rather than the bad.

Ask for assistance. You can reduce your stress by talking to loved ones. Reducing your stress level is another benefit of enlisting the aid of others in trying times.

Chapter 5

EXCESSIVE STRESS AND ANXIETY ABOUT THE FUTURE

Although it may seem useful to worry about the future, doing so is likely to do more harm than good. A future-oriented mindset might help you take charge of your workday and get closer to your objectives, but it also comes with an unspoken drawback.

WHY IS IT THAT WE FEAR WHAT MAY COME

In the face of ambiguity, the body responds with stress. It's natural to be anxious about the future when we're in an unfamiliar position or confronted with baffling obstacles. These emotions serve as guides, preparing us for what is ahead and sometimes inspiring us to take action. When managed properly, stress can have positive effects.

However, our emotional and physical health may begin to suffer when stress becomes chronic.

Too much worry can also lead to avoiding the same things that stress us out, which can have a multiplicative effect on our anxiety.

People who worry excessively may also have a skewed view of reality. They could act more defensively when confronted with actual or imagined dangers because they expect bad things to happen more frequently.

Although looking forward might help you take charge of your workday and get you closer to your goals, it does come with a drawback that we tend to overlook. Everybody knows that thinking ahead can lead to anxiety about the future.

While it's good to be interested in what the future holds, it's just as vital that you stop worrying about it if it's getting in the way of your present activities.

WHEN WE FRET TOO MUCH ABOUT THE FUTURE, WE RISK LOSING THESE THREE THINGS

Being unable to enjoy the here and now.

You can't enjoy life in the present if you spend all your time fretting about the future. Because of this, you can't concentrate on the task at hand and won't get very far. You need to get on this right away. If you don't, you'll waste a lot of mental and physical resources obsessing over hypothetical threats that will never materialize.

Instead, you should give some thought to starting a meditation practice or incorporating mindfulness habits into your daily life. This will allow you to worry less about the future and enjoy life more in the here and now.

THE FIRE IS OUT

Many of us don't realize we're burning out until it's too late, despite the fact that the warning indicators are rather evident. If you're always worried about what the future holds, you can miss the warning signs that things are about to get much worse.

Take a deep breath and consider what you can do today to stop the downward spiral into burnout. It may be as easy as getting a new set of applications or finding ways to make your day job more like a vacation.

FINDING IT IMPOSSIBLE TO STRIKE A HEALTHY WORK LIFE BALANCE

Worrying about the future makes it harder to strike a good work-life balance, which we all seek. Focusing on external factors can make us forget about the inside ones.

This is why I stress the importance of identifying one's unique sweet spot to my clients. Once individuals begin to function from that space, they will more readily position themselves in the path of chances that support their goals and bring more balance to their lives.

Now that you have more of an excuse to quit fretting over the future, you can concentrate on finding ways to make the most of the here and now. When you succeed, you'll be free to pursue any goals you set for yourself.

We can nearly always trace the origins of our worries back to the unknowns of the future. The worry that one's ambitions and hopes may remain unfulfilled is often brought to light.

But that's no reason to give up on your aspirations and hopes in an effort to reduce your anxiety. In order to stay motivated and focused on the future, it is essential to define long-term objectives and dreams. It's easy to lose focus and motivation if you don't have anything to work toward.

However, future concerns can overshadow the present if you can't stop thinking about them. And this way of life can be rather damaging.

After all, tomorrow holds anything at all. There are just too many possible outcomes and paths to take into account to ever feel like you have a firm grasp on the situation.

Worry is exacerbated when one overgeneralizes, or extrapolates, from the present to the future. Extrapolating the difficulties of the present into an identical forecast of the future might lead to a constant state of anxiety.

Worrying nonstop, though, is something you can put an end to. You can feel more grounded and at peace with the help of these three anxiety-busting techniques.

CONDENSE THE FUTURE INTO BITE-SIZED PIECES

Your inability to quit worrying about the future is evidenced by the fact that you are allowing yourself to make lists of bad things that could happen and how much agony you would feel as a result. If you continue down this path, you risk undermining your current efforts.

Think about the "one day at a time" credo of Alcoholics Anonymous so you don't get discouraged and give up on your objectives and goals. Today, that is all that matters.

This is the method my client Paula used to complete a half marathon. She tried to take things one minute at a time whenever she felt like giving up. There were times when she doubted her ability to continue, but she promised herself that she would at least keep going for one minute.

You can increase your ability to deal with various stresses by training yourself to deal with them one day at a time, one minute at a time, and one breath at a time.

Change your perspective and train yourself to think both globally and locally.

One of my friends constantly shifts his point of view in order to deal with his chronic anxiety about the future. To overcome obstacles, he looks at the big picture, which is usually a more admirable objective. Because the end outcome, the broad picture, is so terrifying, he tries to keep his attention on the specifics at hand.

Focusing on the here and now will reveal what is immediately accessible and in your power. Few of us feel in charge of what will happen decades from now, but most of us can see clearly what we can influence in the here and now. What we need to do in the next five minutes, hour, or day is easy to picture in our minds, but what lies beyond that is more difficult to imagine. It's easy to become lost in the abstract details and feel paralyzed by anxiety about the future.

SEEK THE CAUSE, NOT THE EFFECT

Try re-framing your anxiety and doubt about the future as excitement and anticipation. What if your fear of the future is just a hint that you need to shift your attention to something more pressing? What if the anxiety you're feeling is giving you the boost you need to tackle those pressing new projects? Is it possible that your fears are really just a call for you to focus on the future?

Inquiring into such matters helps you take

charge of your worrying. You will no longer feel helpless. Eventually, you'll begin to feel more confident in your abilities.

Having some distance from a problem is helpful for gaining perspective and channeling your anxiety into action. Perspectives can be swiftly and drastically altered by asking probing questions like those above.

These three techniques are among the most effective for putting an end to anxious thoughts. They are effective because they bring attention back to the here and now, rather than the uncertainties of the future. And when you give your full attention to the here and now, you experience a sense of peace and well-being. The ability to direct your own life's trajectory returns, allowing you to finally master your fears.

Chapter 6

AFFECTIVE DISORDERS OR ANXIETY RELYING EXCESSIVELY ON ONE'S MEMORIES

Anxiety disorders are classified as a mental illness. Suffering from anxiety makes daily tasks challenging. Nervousness, panic, and terror, accompanied by profuse sweating and a racing heart, are classic symptoms. Medication and cognitive behavioral therapy are both effective treatments.

DO ANXIOUS THOUGHTS FORCE YOU TO REPLAY THE PAST OVER AND OVER

When people ruminate, they dwell excessively on a topic or incident in their lives. It has been said that "rumination is the act of thinking over and over again about things that have already happened and cannot be changed." If you tend to be anxious or are one of those persons, you may be more susceptible to this than others.

WHY DO PEOPLE FEEL ANXIOUS

Anxiety disorders rarely emerge or have a single, identifiable cause. Personality, stressful events, and health all play a part.

PROBLEMS IN MENTAL HEALTH THAT RUN IN THE FAMILY

Anxiety disorders may run in families, and some people may be born with a tendency to develop them. Having a parent or close relative with anxiety or another mental health illness does not, however, increase your risk of developing anxiety to the same degree.

ELEMENTA DE PERSONALIA

Evidence suggests that some personality features increase the risk of developing anxiety. Anxiety can develop in children and young people who, for example, strive for perfection, are easily startled or embarrassed, are very reserved or shy, have low self-esteem, or have a need to exert excessive control over their surroundings.

CHRONIC SOURCES OF TENSION

One or more stressful life events may contribute to the development of anxiety disorders. Common precipitants consist of:

employment insecurity or a desire for a promotion

Shift in living quarters

pregnancy, labor, and delivery

difficulties in the home and in interpersonal relationships

severe emotional shock caused by exposure to stress or trauma

trauma or abuse, verbal, sexual, physical, or emotional

loss of a loved one through death.

ILLNESSES OF A PHYSICAL NATURE

Anxiety disorders and the treatment of anxiety or physical sickness can both be influenced by chronic physical illness. Anxiety disorders are commonly accompanied by a number of chronic illnesses, such as diabetes, asthma heart illness with high blood pressure Physiological issues, such as an overactive thyroid, can manifest in ways that are similar to anxiety. Going to the doctor to get checked out in case your anxiety has a physical basis is a good idea.

DISTINCTIVE PSYCHIATRIC DISORDERS

Others may experience several anxiety disorders or other mental health illnesses, while some people may only experience one. There is a strong correlation between depression and anxiety disorders. All of these issues should be screened for simultaneously and treated accordingly.

SUBSTANCE ABUSE

In order to cope with their worry, some people turn to drugs and alcohol. There is a possibility that this contributes to the dual diagnosis of substance abuse and anxiety in some circumstances. Anxiety disorders can become worse after drinking or using drugs, as the effects of the substance begin to wear off. In addition to addressing the underlying mental health issue, it is crucial to screen for and treat any substance use disorders that may be present.

SOME FACTS ABOUT ANXIETY THAT MAY HELP YOU FOCUS

Although we humans are hardwired to be vigilant in the face of potential threats, the constant barrage of data is causing an increase in stress and anxiety that is beginning to have a negative impact on our ability to function normally. Many of us have a hard time stopping our thoughts from racing ahead, fixating on what might go wrong, or back, ruminating on what has gone wrong. For this reason, putting an end to the practice of time travel would be a significant move toward relieving our worries.

Perhaps the concept of physically traveling across time is more commonly discussed in science fiction. However, throughout the majority of the day, our minds are physically moving from one point in time to another. Our thoughts might easily go to the past or the future at any given time. To learn, develop, progress, and gain knowledge, this method is essential. However, most of our worry stems from our incessant preoccupation with the past that we cannot change and the future that we cannot predict. Here are five facts about anxiety that, if understood, can help us live in the here and now with far less worry.

WHEN PEOPLE FEEL ANXIOUS THEY FREQUENTLY WORRY ABOUT THE FUTURE

Anticipation is a major source of worry for humans. Uncertainty is one of life's constants, and it can be a major source of worry and anxiety. Despite the fact that our fears of the future can feel like arrows being shot at us, anxiety can also serve as a peculiar sort of protection. No one here is sure they can survive without it. In some ways, it may feel inseparable from our very selves. On some level, we may even justify our worry by telling ourselves that we'll be better able to handle whatever it is we're afraid of if we just think about it or plan for it ahead of time.

Some of us even believe that anxiety safeguards us from the future, usually in the form of the erroneous idea that our darkest worries may be prevented if we worry about them enough. We rehearse tragedy and tell ourselves terrible stories in an attempt to control the uncontrollable or be confident about ambiguity, but to what end? Getting ahead of ourselves is a certain way to lose our minds. We aren't experiencing reality or even the present moment.

THE PAST IS A POSSIBLE ORIGIN OF ANXIETY

We all mentally relive stressful or regretful experiences, but some people get locked in a loop of reliving the same events over and over again. Implicit memories, things we don't necessarily remember consciously but that have shaped our thoughts, feelings, and behaviors, are only one manner in which this occurs.

Conflicts from the past might reawaken in us in response to many different situations in the here and now. We are more likely to feel anxious when we are confronted with situations that cause us to relive painful emotions or recall the "critical inner voices" we have about ourselves or our lives. For this and other reasons, deciphering our past can be a potent resource for figuring out and conquering our present-day anxieties. Stress at work or in a relationship may appear to be based on immediate factors, but how we actually respond, feel, and torment ourselves in these situations is often a mirror of long-simmering emotions.

ANXIETY MIGHT BE EXACERBATED BY ONE'S OWN CRITICAL THOUGHTS

The critical inner voice is a detrimental thought process that criticizes, undermines, and improperly advises us based on unhealthy, damaging messaging we picked up at an early age. Anxiety can be amplified by this self-critical thought process.

We can let our inner critic, who often causes us anxiety, impair our performance at work. We consider the worst-case scenarios and think things like:

You need to do this right or you'll look foolish in front of everyone.

Seeing as how everything is starting to pile up, you should have worked all weekend. It's impossible for you to finish in time.

This is too big of a project for you to handle alone. You fail miserably as a messenger. No one thinks highly of you.

Really, you have everyone duped. You simply cannot proceed in this manner. You will be let go from your current position.

Our connections suffer when we think things like:

The plan is certain to fail. Put your expectations in check. Maintain a safe distance.

No longer does she have any real affection for you. The question is, "Where did you go wrong?" In other words, you need to figure it out.

At this point, if you don't grab his interest, you'll lose him.

Because of you, it's ruined, and now he or she will never accept you.

Our role as parents is impacted:

Your kids will probably grow up to despise you because of how terrible a parent you will be.

It seems you can't even care for your own child. It's completely beyond your ken to act.

You're really screwing them over as a parent because of all the mistakes you've made.

You assumed you'd turn out differently from your parents, but you're actually turning out to be just like them!

Whatever is happening in our lives is made much worse and more anxious by the commentary of our inner critic. The good news is that we can feel considerably stronger in ourselves, more rooted in reality, and a lot less stressed when we recognize and challenge our critical inner voice. To confront this pessimistic outlook head-on can paradoxically cause us to feel nervous at first. However, this is a healthy sort of worry that indicates we are developing and evolving.

Eventually, as we continue to recognize and release our critical inner voice, we can experience more serenity and safety within ourselves, as we are less likely to be scared, anxious, or triggered by this internal foe. Instead, we are becoming more attuned to its occurrence and learning that its messages are neither truthful nor helpful and are largely responsible for our uneasiness.

ANXIETY CAN BE CONQUERED AT LAST

We are not obligated to maintain a link to our dreadful history or a bleak vision of our potential future. Allowing ourselves to disconnect from the outside world and focus on ourselves and the here and now is one way to halt time-traveling and enjoy life more fully. To alleviate anxiety, we can employ tried-and-true methods like focusing on our breath and reawakening our senses.

Most significantly, we may argue with that part of our mind that is always picking holes in our ideas. There are concrete actions we can take to combat this critical voice within. Assuming we can master this "voice," we will be able to take on more. If we can get some distance, we can practice self-kindness. Thoughts appear to us as what they really are: merely thoughts, existing independently of ourselves and the world around us. When our inner critic starts to take over our thoughts, we can be gentle with ourselves and bring ourselves back to the present moment.

"If you want to conquer the anxiety of life, live in the moment, live in the breath," says Amit Ray, a mindfulness teacher. Probably the hardest part will be allowing ourselves to take that step.

Chapter 7

RAPID ADAPTATION TO PRESSURED CONDITIONS IS A HALLMARK OF STRESS

That's because the reaction is the body's defense mechanism against stress. There are repercussions on the endocrine, respiratory, cardiovascular, and nervous systems. Stress can increase heart rate, breathing rate, perspiration, and muscle tension. As a bonus, it may provide a jolt of energy.

STRESS... WHAT IS IT

The body's natural reaction to any demand or threat is stress. The "fight-or-flight" reaction, often called the "stress response," is a quick, instinctive process in which the body's defenses go into high gear in response to perceived or actual danger.

To put it simply, the stress reaction is your body trying to keep you safe. Once it's functioning properly, it aids in maintaining mental clarity, physical stamina, and alertness. Stress can be lifesaving in dangerous situations, giving you the strength to fight off an attacker or the impulse to slam on the brakes to escape a collision.

The ability to rise to the occasion is one benefit of stress. What makes you stay alert during a professional presentation, focus intently as you shoot a game-winning free throw, or force yourself to study when you'd rather be watching TV is the ability to maintain a high level of motivation. While some degree of stress can be beneficial, too much of it can have negative consequences for your health, outlook, productivity, relationships, and overall quality of life.

If you frequently experience feelings of stress

and anxiety, it is essential to take steps toward restoring equilibrium to your nervous system. Learning to recognize the signs and symptoms of chronic stress and taking action to decrease its adverse effects can help protect you from its negative impacts and improve your mood and outlook.

CONSEQUENCES OF PERSISTENT ANXIETY

In terms of your neurological system, it has a hard time telling the difference between emotional and physical dangers. A fight with a buddy, an impending deadline at work, or a stack of unpaid bills can all cause your body to respond as strongly as if you were in a real life-or-death crisis. However, the more frequently you engage your emergency stress system, the less control you will have over its subsequent activation.

We live in a demanding society, and if you're like many of us, you may find that your body is constantly in a state of stress. Also, that can cause some major health issues. Chronic stress can cause problems for almost every bodily function. It lowers resistance to disease, disrupts digestion and reproduction, raises blood pressure and cholesterol levels, and accelerates the aging process. It can really alter neural pathways in the brain, making you more susceptible to issues like anxiety, depression, and other mental health disorders.

Here are some of the health issues that can be attributed to stress or that stress can exacerbate:

SUFFERING FROM LOW MOOD OR ANXIETY

Any form of pain

Disturbed sleep

Illnesses caused by the body's immune system attacking itself

Issues with digestion

Eczema and other skin disorders

Infectious illness of the heart

Issues with Weight

Problems with reproduction

Issues with concentration and recall

Indicators that your stress levels are through the roof

The silent, sneaking nature of stress is its greatest threat. The truth is, you can learn to live with it. It becomes used to the point of normalcy. Although it is having a significant impact on you, you are oblivious to it. This is why it's so crucial to recognize the early indicators of stress overload before it's too late.

BRAIN PROBLEMS

Challenges Keeping Memories Alive

Poor focus

Poor discretion

having a pessimistic outlook

Worrying or restless thinking

Restless fretting

PSYCHOLOGICAL SYMPTOMS

Suffering with melancholy or a persistent bad mood

Fear and restlessness

dispositions of irritation, anger, or sadness

Overwhelmed with stress

Isolation and loneliness

Alternate conditions of emotional or mental health

SYMPTOMS IN YOUR BODY

Discomfort and pain

Either diarrhea or constipation

Headaches, nausea, and fainting have been reported.

discomfort in the chest and a racing heart

Absence of sexual desire

Common cold and flu symptoms

PROBLEMS WITH BEHAVIOR

Increasing or decreasing one's caloric intake

Insufficient or excessive slumber

Isolating oneself from social contact

Putting off or avoiding one's duties

Reducing stress via intoxication

Anxious routines

THE ORIGINS OF TENSION

Stressors are the conditions and demands that contribute to an individual's heightened state of emotional arousal. Most of the time, when we think about stress, we picture something terrible, like a demanding job or a tense romantic relationship. But anything that calls for a lot of effort on your part might be stressful.

Successes like this can be anything from getting married to buying a house to graduating from college to finding a new job.

Not all stressful situations have an outside cause. One's own thoughts and beliefs can also be a source of stress, especially if they lead one to be overly anxious about the future or to view life through a negative lens.

Finally, how you interpret a stressful situation is a major factor. What stresses you out may not even phase another person; they may even find it enjoyable. Some of us would rather die than act or speak in public, yet others thrive under the bright lights. When the stakes at work are too high, some people respond well to further strain while others shut down. And while you may take pleasure in pitching in to assist take care of your parents as they age, your siblings may find the responsibility of caregiving to be too much to bear.

HERE ARE SOME EXAMPLES OF COMMON STRESSORS IN THE OUTSIDE WORLD

Upheavals in one's life

Tasks or studies

Conflict in relationships

Difficulties in obtaining sufficient funds

For lack of time

Family and young ones

INTRINSIC SOURCES OF STRESS FREQUENTLY ENCOUNTERED IN DAILY LIFE INCLUDE

Pessimism

Incapacity to tolerate ambiguity

lack of flexibility in thought processes

Disappointing internal dialogue

Impossible standards of excellence

No-holds-barred mentality

WHAT CAUSES YOU THE MOST ANXIETY

There are strategies you can employ to deal with whatever is causing you stress and get back on track. Common causes of anxiety in daily living include:

ANXIETY CAUSED BY WORK

While some degree of stress at the office is to be expected, experiencing chronic or severe stress can have negative effects on your physical and mental health, your relationships, and your quality of life at home. Workplace success or failure may even depend on it. You may shield yourself from the negative impacts of stress, increase your job happiness, and fortify your well-being in and out of the office regardless of your goals or the nature of your profession.

THE PSYCHOLOGICAL TOLL OF JOBLESSNESS

The loss of a job can be a very trying situation. It is natural to experience negative emotions such as anger, hurt, depression, grief over losses, and worry about the future. The sudden and drastic nature of job loss and unemployment can be devastating to one's sense of stability and identity. Although the pressure may be too much to bear, there are many things you can do to emerge from this trying time more powerful, resilient, and with a clearer sense of direction.

PRESSURE FROM THE BANK ACCOUNT

We're all struggling financially right now, people from all walks of life and all corners of the globe. One of the most prevalent sources of stress in modern life is concern about money, whether due to the loss of a job, mounting debt, unanticipated costs, or some other issue. There are, however, strategies available for coping with the current economic climate, reducing anxiety, and regaining financial footing.

131

RETIREMENT

As much as you may be looking forward to it, retirement is not without its share of challenges. At first glance, being free from your regular routine and lengthy commute may sound like a dream come true. After a while, though, you might miss the routine and routinely-scheduled days that employment provided, as well as the companionship that came from interacting with others at the office. There are effective strategies for adjusting to retirement and dealing with the stress that comes with it.

STRAIN ON CAREGIVERS

Providing care for another person can be demanding, especially if you feel like you're in over your head or have little say in the matter. Unmanaged caregiver stress can have negative effects on physical health, interpersonal connections, and mental well-being, ultimately leading to burnout. But there are many things you can do to lessen the burden of caregiving and rediscover the balance, joy, and hope that you once had.

LOSS AND SORROW

Losing someone or something you care about deeply is incredibly difficult to deal with. The anguish and pressure brought on by a loss can often be too much to bear. It's possible that you'll feel a wide range of negative and unexpected feelings, from shock and rage to disbelief, remorse, and deep sadness. While there is no set formula for dealing with loss, there are methods that have been shown to be helpful in reducing emotional distress and paving the way for individuals to accept their loss, discover meaning in it, and move on with their lives.

WHEN DOES STRESS BECOME HARMFUL

Recognizing your individual stress threshold is crucial due to the far-reaching effects of stress. To what extent, however, stress becomes unhealthy, varies from person to person. Some people seem to be able to take everything life throws at them, while others easily give up or become bitter when faced with even minor setbacks. The adrenaline rush of a high-pressure existence may even bring out the best in some people.

SOME OF THE THINGS THAT CAN AFFECT HOW WELL YOU HANDLE STRESS ARE

This is the group that will always have your back. Having a group of caring friends and family members behind you can be a huge stress reliever. The burdens of daily life ease when you have reliable friends and family to lean on. Conversely, the higher your danger of **stress breakdown when you're lonely and alone.**

A feeling of being in charge. You can deal with stress better if you have faith in yourself and your ability to affect outcomes and stick with problems. However, if you believe that you are helpless in the face of adversity and that your life is largely determined by other factors, stress is more likely to derail you.

What you're thinking and how you see the world. How you frame life's unavoidable difficulties can have a significant impact on how well you deal with stress. Having a positive outlook and expecting the best will make you more resilient. People who are better able to handle stress are those who are optimistic in the face of adversity, can laugh at themselves, have faith in a greater cause, and realize that change is a constant.

How well you are able to control your feelings. Stress and agitation are more likely to occur if you are unable to soothe and calm yourself in times of emotional distress, such as when you are feeling sad, angry, or troubled. Increase your stress tolerance and improve your resilience by learning to recognize and manage your feelings.

It all comes down to your foresight and planning. Understanding the nature and duration of a stressful event can help you better manage it. For instance, if you have a reasonable expectation of how quickly you'll be able to recover from surgery, the discomfort of the recovery period won't be as difficult to bear.

BUILDING A STRONGER STRESS RESISTANCE

The time has come to act. You can immediately begin to feel better by increasing your amount of physical exercise, which can help you feel less stressed. Getting your body moving on a regular basis can help you feel better emotionally and mentally, providing a welcome diversion from the stresses that can otherwise build up. Walking, running, swimming, and dancing are all great examples of rhythmic movements that, when performed consciously, can have a significant impact on health (focusing your attention on the physical sensations you experience as you move).

Make friends and associates. When you're feeling tense or insecure, talking to another person face to face can release hormones that calm you down. A little moment of kindness from another person, in the form of words or a friendly glance, can have a profound effect on your state of mind. Therefore, surround yourself with positive people and don't let your responsibilities prevent you from having fun.

Make it a top goal to cultivate deeper and more fulfilling relationships if you currently lack them or if your interpersonal interactions are causing you stress.

TAKE ADVANTAGE OF YOUR SENSES

Involving your senses (sight, hearing, taste, smell, touch, and movement) is a quick approach to reduce stress. To succeed, you must determine which kind of sensory stimulation are most beneficial. When you listen to an inspiring song, do you feel more at peace? Is it the aroma of freshly ground coffee, for instance? Maybe touching an animal helps you feel more grounded and in the present moment. The ideal way to process sensory information is one that you discover through trial and error; everyone reacts to stimuli slightly differently.

MASTER THE ART OF UNWINDING

Although stress is unavoidable, you can manage its impact on your life. The relaxation reaction is triggered by practices like yoga, meditation, and deep breathing, and it's the opposite of the stress response since it induces a mood of calm and ease. Regular participation in such pursuits has been shown to have positive effects on both mental and physical health. They help you maintain composure even when things get hectic.

MAINTAIN A NUTRITIOUS DIET.

What you put into your body has a direct impact on how you feel emotionally and how well you can handle the stresses of daily life. Fresh fruit and vegetables, high-quality protein, and omega-3 fatty acids might help you better cope with life's ups and downs, whereas a diet full of processed and convenience food, refined carbohydrates, and sugary snacks can increase stress symptoms.

SOOTHE YOUR WEARY BONES AND SLEEP IT OFF

Being overly fatigued might make you act erratically, which can only add to your stress levels. Simultaneously, constant anxiety might make it difficult to fall asleep. Sleeping better can help you feel less stressed, more productive, and emotionally balanced, whether you're having difficulties falling asleep or staying asleep at night.

Chapter 8

INJURIES TO THE MIND

Varying degrees of mental trauma can be just as incapacitating as physical ones, so it's important to get professional help if you've suffered one. Post-traumatic stress disorder depression, adjustment disorders, anxiety, and specific phobias are among the most frequent kinds of psychological harm.

PSYCHIATRIC WOUNDS

Many clients in personal injury cases suffer both physical and emotional harm. Especially after car accidents, victims of psychological trauma may exhibit incapacitating symptoms including flashbacks, insomnia, anxiety, or phobias, all of which are frequently disregarded.

Bond Turner is familiar with the nuances of both primary and subsequent psychological injury. Including accountants, interpreters, and barristers, our team of 45 Grade A solicitors and Chartered Legal Executives has successfully pursued multi-million pound claims on behalf of clients who have suffered catastrophic injuries.

HOW DOES ONE SUFFER A MENTAL WOUND

It's easy to forget about the victim's mental health when physical wounds are so severe. Depending on the nature of the damage, the effects of a mental trauma might be just as incapacitating as those of a physical one, necessitating specialized care.

depression, adjustment problems, anxiety, and specific phobias are the most frequent manifestations of psychological trauma. Our team can arrange for a psychiatrist and psychologist to evaluate the extent of any mental injury and provide appropriate therapy, and rehabilitation can help get you there.

Injuries of the mind are becoming an increasing issue for businesses. The goal of any company should be to provide a stress-free environment where employees may thrive. The first step in protecting yourself from psychological harm is realizing what causes it. Lost time and productivity, as well as potential workers' compensation claims, can add up quickly when a worker suffers a psychological injury. While the laws in Australia are complicated, if your mental illness was brought on by your job, Workcover may pay for your medical expenses.

WHAT DOES PSYCHOLOGICAL HARM IMPLY

Psychological trauma is characterized by cognitive or emotional symptoms that have a significant negative effect on a person's daily functioning. Depression, post-traumatic stress disorder, and anxiety are all examples of psychological damage.

A combination of environmental, organizational, and personal variables can lead to psychological harm on the job. There is loud machinery, dangerous chemicals, and accidents.

Some of the issues that might arise in an organization are a lack of leadership support, a lack of stability, and an overwhelming amount of pressure. A person's susceptibility to sustaining a mental health damage depends on their unique personality and life events. Poor psychological safety has been demonstrated to be expensive for Australian firms.

The term "secondary psychological injury" refers to the psychological harm that occurs as a result of the One's mental health can suffer secondary damage if they've already sustained a physical wound. Depression, despair, rage, disturbed sleep, and decreased motivation and engagement are just some of the secondary issues that might arise after an employee suffers a physical injury. Persistent suffering, reliance on medication, and separation from loved ones and coworkers can exacerbate these mental health problems.

CAUSES AND INSTANCES OF PSYCHOLOGICAL HARM

typical sources of workplace tension that put employees at risk for suffering mental harm.

STRESS OVER UNCERTAINTY OF EMPLOYMENT

Employees' mental and physical health might be negatively impacted by the constant prospect of organizational reorganizations, mergers, and redundancies. Stress from a lack of job security has been linked to worse health outcomes than both smoking and high blood pressure. More and more people are working in precarious, low-paying jobs where they could be let go at any time without notice or compensation.

If their contract is terminated, some people worry that they won't be able to make ends meet. They may be concerned about the opinion of their manager and the company's plans for their long-term employment. Stress from this situation can build up over the course of years, causing significant mental health problems.

Due to the lack of access to contractors may be less likely to seek professional psychiatric or psychological care than permanent employees Some people worry about losing their jobs if they take time off, and this is exacerbated by the lack of paid leave benefits.

Many employees may not view job instability as a significant source of stress or emotional harm due to the fact that people's perspectives vary. Some people are willing to forego employment stability in exchange for the increased hourly pay and bonus rates that come with casual labor. They have full faith that they can easily find another employment and avoid financial hardship if their current one were to end.

The best way to avoid becoming a victim of work insecurity is to look for a position that provides more stability than your current one. It's true that there's no such thing as a "forever job," but you might be happier in a full-time one.

TOO MUCH WORK

Staff members are typically pushed to multitask more during tough economic times. No one is ever replaced when they leave or go on vacation, thus the rest of the team must always step up to cover for them. Stress from having to do more at work could lead to decreased productivity, emotional instability, and trouble sleeping, among other negative outcomes.

Some businesses push their employees to the brink of stress and inadequacy by setting goals that are just unattainable. People may find it difficult to unwind and relax after work because of the stress and hectic pace of their daily lives.

Avoid this by communicating your inability to handle the workload with your superiors or asking a coworker to take on some of the work you can't get to.

ACTS OF HARASSMENT AND AGGRESSION TOWARD OTHERS

Workplace bullying can affect adults just as much as it does children in the schoolyard. Bullying in the workplace can take many forms, including words, actions, relationships, and even thoughts. Bullying can manifest itself in a wide variety of ways, including name-calling, social exclusion, sexual harassment, mental games, meaningless assignments, hazing, initiations, threats, physical violence, and accidents. Workplace bullying can occur at any workplace can involve a management, coworker, or group of people.

Victims of bullying may suffer from increased levels of stress, anxiety, and depression; they may also lose self-esteem and motivation at work.

Workers' compensation claims for emotional harm sustained as a result of bullying at work can be expensive for businesses. A QLD mine worker with adjustment disorder, anxiety, and social phobia was awarded "significant" damages earlier this year following a legal struggle with his previous employer.

Avoiding This: It is the responsibility of every employer to ensure that their workplace is free from bullying and harassment. If you ever feel threatened or intimidated on the job, you should tell your boss about it so they can take appropriate action.

PROBLEMATIC CLIENT MANAGEMENT

Staff members who have to deal with irate clients may continue to feel stressed long after the issue has been resolved and the consumer has departed. The lasting effects of an incident on a worker can be much more detrimental than the occurrence itself. When a situation cannot be solved and a consumer cannot be reassured, it is normal for those involved to experience dread and tension. They fret over whether or not they will be able to deal effectively with the following challenge.

What stresses out one worker greatly may be something else entirely, just as how one person views job instability may be something else entirely to another. Employees have varying reactions to dealing with challenging consumers.

Some workers have the humility to know they can't help everyone. They know that even an irate client is forgotten after they have given their all to the job. They are dedicated to enhancing the quality of their client encounters. Something that would seriously affect the mental health of one worker might not affect the mind of another.

If you find that dealing with irate or difficult customers causes undue stress and anxiety, it may be beneficial to inquire about training options with your company. Confidence in handling future incidents can be gained via preparation and familiarity with existing resources and procedures.

WORK ROTATION

There has been extensive research into the health risks associated with night and shift employment. It is now widely accepted that working late can lead to everything from an increased risk of cancer to a weakened immune system and even premature death. Recent research has focused on the mental health implications of working shifts, and it has found that they can be as detrimental as the physical ones.

Increased stress and discontentment are the results of shift workers' circadian rhythms being disrupted. One research of nurses in the United Kingdom found that working shifts was associated with lower levels of job satisfaction. Night shift nurses had greater physiological and emotional distress, leading to decreased job satisfaction.

Negative effects on mental health have been linked to shift work, and the stress of missing out on family obligations and social engagements can compound the negative effects of working irregular hours.

If your shift schedule is causing you stress, discuss the issue with your supervisor and see if you can cut back on your night shifts or look for a different line of work that doesn't necessitate as much shift work.

Returns to work following psychological injuries are typically longer than those following physical ones. Treating mental health issues effectively requires early intervention. Alternate career opportunities and conflict resolution are two ways to lessen the likelihood of a long-term mental harm.

HOW TO RECOVER FROM EMOTIONAL WOUNDS

If you have suffered emotional scars, have you ever questioned whether or not you might ever fully recover? Is it possible to recover from severe emotional wounds such as trauma, social exclusion, despair, or a shattered heart.

Maybe you've been in pain for a while, and it just isn't going away.

Maybe you feel helpless, like you've exhausted all possible options.

Or maybe you think it's too late or you're too old to make a change.

When you're feeling down and out, it's hard to imagine how you'll ever be able to pick yourself up and start over. There's nothing wrong with questioning whether or not you can actually experience emotional healing.

IT IS POSSIBLE TO RECOVER FROM EMOTIONAL TRAUMA

If you are feeling emotionally broken, please know that recovery is possible. As a therapist, I've witnessed countless miraculous comebacks, with patients gaining health, happiness, and a deeper sense of themselves in ways they never thought possible.

True, not everyone can regain their mental equilibrium. For some, the anguish never ends, and they keep on engaging in destructive patterns of thought, feeling, and action.

After working as a therapist and social worker for over two decades, I have observed several patterns among those who are able to overcome their emotional trauma and pain. I pray that these musings and suggestions can aid in your own recovery as well.

COUNSELING ADVICE FOR MENDING BROKEN HEARTS

Attempt to accomplish something in small, manageable chunks. Making too many adjustments at once can cause problems. Setting unachievable goals might lead to feelings of frustration and disappointment. And abrupt shifts are usually not maintainable. Making micro-changes, or small, controllable, incremental improvements, might give you the confidence, optimism, and support you need to get better. Here you will find further information regarding the introduction of minor adjustments.

You don't need a complete recovery to feel better; even a partial one would help. It's a common misconception that in order to increase the quality of your life, you need to heal every aspect of your emotional health. This notion, once again, can be depressing and daunting. First and foremost, it's not true. Healing, even slight healing, will enhance the quality of your life. Little by little, you will feel better in terms of your overall disposition, resilience in the face of setbacks, interpersonal interactions, sense of self-worth, and capacity to carry out your daily tasks.

ATTEMPT TO ACCOMPLISH SOMETHING IN SMALL MANAGEABLE CHUNKS

Making too many adjustments at once can cause problems. Setting unachievable goals might lead to feelings of frustration and disappointment. And abrupt shifts are usually not maintainable. Making micro-changes, or small, controllable, incremental improvements, might give you the confidence, optimism, and support you need to get better. Here you will find further information regarding the introduction of minor adjustments.

THE PROCESS OF HEALING IS NOT BINARY

A little bit of healing is likely to make a big difference in your life. It's a common misconception that in order to increase the quality of your life, you need to heal every aspect of your emotional health. This notion, once again, can be depressing and daunting. First and foremost, it's not true. Healing, even slight healing, will enhance the quality of your life. Little by little, you will feel better in terms of your overall disposition, resilience in the face of setbacks, interpersonal interactions, sense of self-worth, and capacity to carry out your daily tasks.

HAVE PERSISTENCE AND PATIENCE

A lot of effort goes into healing. Be patient and give yourself time to absorb new information and develop your abilities. And we need to attempt new things, push ourselves in other directions, and keep going even when things get tough.

HAVE A REASONABLE OUTLOOK

When it comes to expectations, I'm a firm believer that more realistic is better. The negative emotions we feel, typically directed at ourselves, prevent us from moving on with our healing when we fail to do so. Predicting that things will always move in a positive direction is one of the most typical examples of wishful thinking I encounter. Nobody just keeps getting healthier and stronger indefinitely. Two steps ahead, and one step back, is more typical of progress than steady advancement. In all candor, you shouldn't be shocked if progress consists of two steps back for every one forward. This is not a setback, but rather a fact. Even if progress is slower and more circuitous than you'd like, it will happen if you keep your sights set on the prize and practice patience, tenacity, and self-compassion along the way.

Think of failures as natural steps along the way and as lessons to be learned. Experiencing a setback is not only inevitable, but also crucial. Our understanding of what does not work can often be more illuminating than that of what works. The best way to move forward and toward greater healing and self-love is to embrace the inevitable nature of setbacks and relapses and to challenge yourself to be curious about what you may learn from them.

Make self-care and kindness to oneself a top priority. A high bar requires a high investment in oneself. It takes a lot of effort, time, and even money to focus on emotional healing. If you want to keep continuing, it's important to tune into your emotions and the sensations in your body (such tight muscles, headaches, weariness, etc.) to learn what it needs. Invest in taking care of yourself and making sure you're heard.

ACCEPT ASSISTANCE WHEN OFFERED

Isolation is counterproductive to the healing process. It takes courage to reach out for assistance, especially if you've been betrayed before. The benefits of seeking out for assistance, however, are numerous, including emotional support, direction, and the ability to overcome shame. Help comes in all shapes and sizes, so I hope you'll consider it an extension of self-care and seek out the assistance that's most suitable for you.

GET SOMEPLACE YOU CAN FEEL SECURE EMOTIONALLY

Emotional wounds are extremely difficult to heal if one does not first feel physically and emotionally protected. When the nervous system has been traumatized or deeply wounded, it is adaptive to remain hypervigilant for threats. The nervous system's overarching goal is security. However, sometimes we seek for indicators of danger so intensively that we miss cues of safety; when this happens, we remain in a high-alert or fight-or-flight state, making it difficult to connect with others, trust, relax, be vulnerable, and regain our equilibrium and well-being. You may begin to recognize situations in which you feel secure, as well as those in which you do not.

There are no people who are immune to emotional pain or who will not experience it at some point in their lives. Some of them we are able to close without any issues, while others appear to be closed, only to reopen at the most inopportune times.

Sometimes life throws us a curveball, and we have to deal with it the best way we know how. Anxiety and other bad feelings build up inside of us as a result of these circumstances. Our ability to control these feelings is not always at our disposal. Because of this, we have put together this manual to help you get through any trying time in your life.

Understanding the nature of emotional wounds and their causes is prerequisite to learning effective treatment options.

Physical wounds heal faster than emotional ones, but both can be caused by traumatic events. These events leave us feeling devastated, enraged, or even terrified. A personal emotional wound can be caused by anything that gives us pain.

Once we've lived through this, we'll have vivid memories of it for years to come. Thus, it is crucial that we discover methods to aid in the management of the feelings it elicits, such as frustration. The path to success is paved with love and mutual appreciation.

One need only reflect back on a time when they felt hurt or wronged to identify an emotional wound. The reality is that hurt feelings can come in many forms.

Chapter 9

FEELINGS OF GUILT AND THEIR ACHE

Although guilt is a mental experience, it can manifest itself physically as tension and discomfort. Feelings of anxiety and discomfort are misinterpreted as guilt because of preoccupation with past transgressions. As a result of associating those ideas with the discomfort, you feel the pain more acutely.

ACCUSATIONS OF NATURAL GUILT

Guilt is a natural emotion to feel if you have done something wrong and are sorry for it. Adaptive guilt is the kind that pushes you to do something about it or make a positive change in your behavior because you know it will help you out in the long run. As an example, you could assuage your conscience by making amends for a wrongdoing or altering your behavior. However, if you don't deal with the consequences of your actions in a healthy way, you could be plagued by feelings of guilt that prevent you from moving on with your life.

INAPPROPRIATE REMORSE

Regrettably, there are occasions when one feels responsible for something that was beyond their control. To provide one example, individuals may harbor regrets over the fact that they did nothing to stop a tragedy they could not have possibly foreseen. They feel remorse, humiliation, and guilt despite the fact that there was really nothing they could have done.

CONSCIOUS GUILT

Thoughts that are bad or improper are normal human experience, but the accompanying guilt is not. They may worry that having "evil" ideas means they will actually act on them or that their secret will be revealed to others.

GUILT FOR JUST BEING THERE:

Guilt of this sort can be convoluted and is typically focused on issues like wrongdoing or failing to live in accordance with one's values. For example, survivorship guilt is a form of existential guilt. It's not uncommon for folks to feel guilty when they're succeeding but someone they care about are struggling. This can arise if you're the sole survivor of a horrific event that wreaks havoc on the lives of others, or if you're the cause of someone else's tragedy while you escape unscathed.

OVERCOMING FEELINGS OF REMORSE AND MOVING FORWARD

For many years, Heather had not spoken to a childhood friend because of a feud that they both refused to let go of out of bitter pride. Heather realized they needed to make peace before her cancer-stricken buddy passed away. She informed me that she wanted to call me, but that there was a harsh corner of her soul that prevented her from doing so. After months of procrastination, she eventually decided to phone her friend, only to find out that her friend had fallen into a coma and was unable to communicate. Heather felt a new wave of remorse washing over her. 'How could I have let my friend die without saying goodbye?' she questioned. I've tried everything, but I simply **can't let it go. My guilt is too great.**

Like Heather, I'm sure a lot of us have sat around for hours on end going over a painful recollection of wrongdoing. Feeling horrible about yourself because you've done something that goes against your principles (guilt) is a fundamentally human experience. Guilt is a normal human emotion. However, there are certain among us who experience more guilt than others, and it's not always because we've done more wrong. Because of this, it is essential to discover the source of your shame and the specific nature of your guilt. The burden of guilt is great. You should not be burdened by feelings of guilt. Identifying the root cause of your emotions of guilt will help you determine the best course of action for eradicating them, whether that involves making amends, processing the situation, or simply moving on.

MANAGING INNATE REMORSE

Let's say you have a pressing and concrete guilt, like denting your friend's lent automobile or fibbing to your partner about where you were last night. You really can't help but feel bad about it; it's in your nature. A symptom of natural guilt is a focus on the here and now, making it easy to identify. Guilt that arises naturally is excruciatingly distressing, particularly when significant harm has resulted. However, local guilt is fixable, even if the act in question was particularly heinous. Repentance is possible. You can seek pardon, make restitution, and commit to alter your ways. The guilt should fade away if the damage is fixed but if it doesn't, read.

Guilt seems to be hard-wired into the nervous system because of the useful purpose it provides. It acts as a warning signal, alerting you to the fact that you're doing unethically so that you can correct your course. If you accidentally bump into a parked automobile, you might feel compelled to call your mom or leave your contact information. Some social scientists argue that natural shame is one of the driving forces behind the development of social safety nets and movements for social justice, and that it stems from our innate capacity for empathy. An unhealthy relationship with guilt results **in excessive self-condemnation. As a substitute, you let them serve as cues for a course correction.**

Phoning your sick friend helps you get over feeling guilty for not calling sooner. When you feel guilty about spending too much, you learn to restrain yourself. If you feel guilty because you participated in a larger wrong, such as racial injustice or the persecution of one group by another, you may try to effect positive social change. And if the source of your guilt is something you can't change, like a working mother's guilt about missing pick-up time, you concentrate on learning to

FORGIVE YOURSELF

But there is a dark side to natural guilt. It becomes a primary tool of parental and social control rather frequently. This is brilliantly illustrated by an ancient joke. Approximately how many Jewish moms does it take to screw in a light bulb? Not a single one: "I'll simply sit here in the dark and not worry about it." However, women of all backgrounds (Jewish and elsewhere) aren't the only ones who use guilt to control their children. Partners and spouses are included. The same is true of spiritual communities and communities of practice, including yoga communities. Have you ever been caught eating salmon and given the guilt trip by a vegan friend? In reality, natural shame may soon become poisonous if it is punished too severely or utilized as a weapon of control. Toxic guilt, the pervasive sense of being "wrong" or flawed in some basic way, is what we experience when this occurs, and it is a condition of constant, mild misery.

CONFRONTING POISONOUS REGRET

Natural guilt, if allowed to sit and grow, can turn toxic. It manifests as an overwhelming sense that something is wrong with your life overall but you can't put your finger on what it is. This form of floating guilt is the most challenging to overcome because it stems from deeply ingrained subconscious habits called samskaras. If you don't know what you did wrong or if you think your wrongdoing is beyond redemption, how can you make amends to yourself or ask for forgiveness.

This sort of guilt appears to be an unexpected by-product of Judeo-Christian tradition, a hangover from the teaching of original sin. Even while they have a lot to say about sin, karma, and how to avoid or purify transgressions, ancient yogic books like the Bhagavad Gita and the Yoga Sutra do not accept generic guilt. But the yogic teachings can still be useful, even though toxic shame isn't usually included in typical lists of yogic impediments. We need to deal with toxic shame not just to lessen the suffering it causes, but also because it attaches itself to every infraction, no matter how small, and causes us to have irrationally awful thoughts and sentiments about ourselves.

There are two common ways in which people suffer poisonous guilt. To begin with, it may already be an ingrained part of your character, a miasmic sensation that occasionally surfaces and makes you feel down or inadequate. Second, it may be sparked by an external factor, such as your own blunders or the suspicions of others. It doesn't take much to set off your toxic guilt load, whether it's a minor misstep at work, a quarrel with your partner, or a phone call from your mother. At its worst, it can make people feel as if they have to constantly watch their every move for fear of revealing their own inherent badness. Therefore, it is crucial to learn to identify toxic shame so that it can no longer serve as an internal motivator.

Roots of toxic guilt are often found in childhood: Guilt that has no rational basis may be the result of, for example, making a mistake that your parents or school made a great deal out of, or of religious upbringing, particularly one which preaches original sin. Some adherents of the notion of reincarnation (the belief that our present circumstances are impacted by patterns created in former lifetimes) view toxic guilt as the karmic residue of actions from prior lives. The Wheel of Sharp Weapons is a Tibetan yoga classic that identifies the sins that have led to modern issues and suggests practices for dealing with them. Some purist yogic activities, such as daily mantra repetition, karma yoga (selfless service), and making offerings, are said to alleviate guilt.

But there's little doubt that specific, unresolved hurt you've caused in this life can also lead to a toxic pile of guilt. Accumulating a considerable quantity of free-flowing guilt is possible when you have built up a few terrible moments of self-betrayal, cheated on a lover or two, or even when you miss to call your parents or get enough regular exercise. In addition, a yogi on the path to enlightenment typically develops a highly discerning moral compass. The more you try to live according to the moral principles of your spiritual path, the less likely you are to give yourself a pass for offensive or destructive actions. However, you might not have completely broken free of your casual and unconscious ways. You do things that aren't good for you or the people around you, even if you know better, and you feel bad about it afterwards. If you are prepared to go deeper, though, you will often discover that your poisonous shame is unrelated to your actions in any meaningful way. That is precisely why it is so poisonous. For someone with chronic feelings of guilt, the prospect of facing the consequences of any particular transgression in the here and now can be terrifying.

CONFRONTING ULTIMATE GUILT

It's also possible that your guilt stems from political or societal concerns. This is the feeling that comes over you when you see caged animals, read about the misery in Zimbabwe, or realize the extreme advantages you have in life. Existential shame is what I'm calling it. There is a legitimate and understandable basis for feelings of existential guilt. Why? Because there is literally no way to live on Earth without negatively affecting someone else in some way, whether it be the owls whose homes were destroyed when trees were cut down to make way for an office park, the plants you crush while hiking, or the fact that your child was given a spot in a great public school while many of your friends' children were denied admission. Many times, even when we're only trying to get by on a bare minimum, our consumption of resources restricts their availability to people who could really need them.

When I was in school, I heard from a wealthy and stunningly attractive woman who had confided in one of my professors that she was struggling with overwhelming feelings of guilt and melancholy. The question "What have you done with your life?" came back from my instructor. Put a bagel on a tree and then leave it there? The captivating koanlike aspect of my teacher's comment has stuck with me for years, but it's the underlying wisdom that has really stuck with me. That woman's guilt complex included elements of existential guilt, and the only way to alleviate existential guilt is to make unconditional contributions to life. We magazine readers, like that woman, enjoy a privileged environment, with access to amenities unavailable to ninety-five percent of the world's population. A sense of existential guilt is understandable and common. The Vedic sages, whose teachings form the basis for all yogic practices, emphasized the importance of paying respect to one's ancestors, the planet, one's instructors, one's higher power, and one's fellow man. Existential guilt sets in when we fail to make good on such obligations.

Many of us haven't been taught the fundamental gestures that reverence the web of life, and this is a symptom of modern liberal society's extreme individualism, fractured families, and consumerist approach toward spirituality. To be clear, I'm not just referring to environmentally conscious actions, but also to acts of kindness, such as hosting dinner parties, feeding the homeless, stray animals, and local spirits, volunteering, donating, and caring for the elderly.

To make matters worse, we often feel responsible for everyone else's suffering when our poisonous guilt gets mixed up with our existential guilt. A good example is my pal Ellen.

Ellen's mother was quite angry and often took out her frustrations on Ellen's sister. Ellen had much compassion for her sister but felt helpless to prevent their mother from making her the scapegoat. Her inability to do anything about the situation made her feel responsible for everyone else's suffering, a form of survivor's guilt. Ellen's inability to save everyone and bring them up to her standards of morality led her to enable depressed friends, fund spiritual con artists, and break her heart.

The first step for Ellen in learning to distinguish between genuine compassion and pointless self-sacrifice was to examine her guilt when it arose, and to determine whether her grief at not fixing the situation was a result of her current circumstances, or a toxic remnant from her past. Once she did that, the aid she provided to others was no longer tainted by guilt. Naturally, it also got considerably more efficient. Sometimes, like Ellen, we can't quite put our finger on the type of shame we're experiencing. Recognizing a distressing emotion as guilt and determining its specific form makes it much more manageable. When we feel guilty, it's because we haven't been living up to our own standards, and it's the kind of thing that calls for an apology and restitution. Forget about your other sins.

RELEASE YOUR GUILT

And this is where one of the greatest blessings of yoga philosophy can be found. For further information on how to deal with guilt in a yoga context, check out The Yogi's Guide to Self-Forgiveness. The yogic tradition can help us feel better about ourselves by teaching us to recognize our inherent goodness. Particularly in Tantric traditions, there is a way of seeing the world in which the very essence of all existence is sacred. The way you feel about your shame will alter dramatically if you start following a spiritual teaching that, rather than saying humans are inherently defective, teaches you to look past your flaws and allows you to recognize your deeper perfection.

In my opinion, the distinction between these two perspectives on who we are is best illustrated by a tale my professor used to tell. Two monasteries previously stood, each one near a sizable metropolis. The monks at one institution taught their students that all humans are corrupt and that strict self-control and penance were the only means to overcome their wicked nature. The kids at the other monastery were taught to have faith in themselves and their own innate virtue. Each of these monasteries had a young man leave for a time because he needed a break from monastic life. They all escaped via different windows in the dorms, caught rides into town, attended parties, and ended up spending the night with prostitutes. When he woke up the next morning, the youngster from the "sinner" monastery was wracked with severe guilt. He told himself, "I've strayed hopelessly off the path." The return trip would be fruitless. He abandoned the monastic life and joined a local gang instead.

The second boy similarly suffered from a hangover upon awakening. On the other hand, he handled the matter in a quite different way. That was less fulfilling than he had hoped. Probably not; that's not something I plan to repeat any time soon. After that he returned to his monastery, sneaked back in through a window, and was reprimanded. When I was in school, I remember my teacher saying that all it takes is one minor mistake to start a downward spiral of sinful behavior. Knowing that at our core we are divine, that we are all Buddhas, as the yoga sages teach, makes it much easier to forgive ourselves for our mistakes and shortcomings. It's also less difficult to alter our ways. Consequently, the true remedy for our troublesome emotions of guilt is to repeatedly acknowledge the light of God's love that brightens our heart.

JUST HOW CAN I HEAL THE EMOTIONAL WOUND CAUSED BY MY OWN GUILT

Check out the original!

The first step in dealing with guilt is understanding what causes it.

It's natural to feel remorse when you realize you've done something wrong, but it's also possible to feel bad about something you didn't do If you make a mistake, admit it, even if it's just to yourself. But it's just as crucial to recognize when you're putting undue blame on yourself for circumstances outside your control.

Guilt is a common human emotion, yet it is often felt for irrational reasons. You may have regrets about ending a relationship with someone who still cares about you or about being successful professionally while your best buddy struggles to obtain gainful employment.

Feelings of guilt can also arise from a perception of falling short of personal or societal expectations. Naturally, this shame does not take into account the work you've put in to overcome the obstacles that have prevented you from reaching your goals.

JUST A FEW OF THE MOST PROMINENT CULPRITS IN TRIGGERING FEELINGS OF GUILT ARE

ability to endure extreme stress or danger internal strife between your principles and your actions health issues, mental or physical any sort of thought or desire that you feel guilty about putting one's own needs first when one thinks one should be concentrating on helping others Who else is making you feel bad all the time? Here you can find advice on how to deal with a guilt trip.

YOU NEED TO SAY YOU'RE SORRY AND TRY TO MAKE THINGS RIGHT

Making amends for wrongdoing often begins with an apology. When you apologize, you show the person you injured that you feel terrible about what you did and that you want to make sure it doesn't happen again.

Since apologies don't always restore shattered trust, you may not receive forgiveness right away.

Apologizing from the heart still aids in recovery, as it allows you to vent your emotions and face the consequences of your actions.

If you wish to make amends with someone, you should.

the importance of your part

Exhibit regret

Don't make up reasons.

humbly seek pardon

TO APOLOGIZE IS TO PROMISE TO DO BETTER IN THE FUTURE

You may regret not being there for your friends and family when they needed you or for not checking in on them often enough. One way to show that you're ready to make amends after offering an apology is to ask, "What can I do to help?" or "How can I be there for you?"

It's possible you won't always be in a position to directly apologize. Try writing a letter if you are unable to contact the person you have offended. Even if they never read your letter of apology, just getting it out there on paper can help.

Perhaps you should apologize to yourself as

well. Keep in mind that no one is perfect, so there's no need in beating yourself up over an honest slip-up.

Make atonement by promising to be kinder to yourself instead than harsher.

TAKE LESSONS FROM HISTORY

You can't fix everything, and sometimes an error might cost you a dear friend or a precious connection. It's very uncommon to feel trapped by the weight of guilt and grief over a loss.

You have to accept what happened in the past before you can go forward. Remembering the past and dwelling on it will not change anything.

Events cannot be changed by imagining alternative outcomes, but lessons learnt can be taken into account in any situation.

What caused the blunder? Try to get to the bottom of what set you off and what emotions may have pushed you over the line.

With hindsight, what would you change Can you reflect on what your behavior revealed about who you are? Do they highlight any particular habits that could use improvement.

SHOW GRATITUDE

Guilt about asking for assistance is prevalent when people are dealing with difficulties, mental anguish, or health issues. Keep in mind that the reason people connect with others is to create a network of caregiving allies.

Just flip the script and picture the outcome. It's only natural to want to be there for your family and friends when they're in distress. You probably don't want them to feel bad about having a hard time too.

Not feeling capable of doing something on your own is very normal. No one was created to go through life on their own.

Instead of beating yourself up when times are tough, practice appreciation by doing the following.

expressing gratitude to loved ones

conveying your gratitude in a tangible way be

sure to thank those who have helped you by mentioning any successes you've had because of their assistance.

vowing to return the favor once they are in a better position to do so

SUBSTITUTE SELF COMPASSION WITH CRITICAL INTERNAL DIALOGUE

Everyone makes blunders now and then; it doesn't make you a bad person if you do.

Self-criticism can get very severe when you're feeling guilty, but telling yourself how terrible of a job you did won't help. The emotional toll of self-punishment is typically much greater than that of any external consequences.

Instead of beating yourself up, consider what you'd tell a buddy who was in your shoes. Maybe you could highlight their accomplishments, highlight their strengths, and express your appreciation for them.

EQUAL CONSIDERATION IS DUE TO YOU

It's difficult to generalize about people and the situations they find themselves in. The blame for the misstep could rest with you and the others, but it could also rest with the others.

Validating your own value can increase self-assurance, allowing you to think more rationally and resist the influence of negative emotions.

KEEP IN MIND THAT REMORSE CAN SERVE A USEFUL PURPOSE

When you've taken a decision that goes against your ideals, feeling guilty might be a useful wake-up call. Don't let it get to you; instead, put it to good use.

Guilt can serve as a useful lens through which to examine and improve upon those aspects of oneself with which one is unhappy.

Perhaps you have a hard time being truthful and someone has caught you in a lie. Perhaps you wish you could spend more time with your loved ones, but other commitments keep getting in the way.

Doing anything to change those conditions can put you on a course that is more in line with your objectives.

Not making an attempt to keep in touch with pals could lead to feelings of guilt, which could motivate you to do so. If you and your spouse both feel that stress is getting in the way of your relationship, try spending one night a week to just the two of you Similarly, it's important to consider the insights guilt might provide about who you are as a person Feeling bad about hurting someone else is a sign of empathy and a lack of malicious intent. If you want to make a difference in your life, you can try to figure out how to stop repeating that error It may be helpful to consult a mental health professional if you have a history of experiencing negative emotions in response to circumstances outside of your control.

GIVE YOURSELF A BREAK

Essential to self-compassion is the ability to forgive oneself. Self-forgiveness is an acknowledgment that you, like any other human being, are capable of making mistakes. Then you can move on with your life and not let that error define you. Simply by being accepting of who you are, flaws and all, you treat yourself with care and compassion.

To forgive oneself, one must do the following four things

Do what you need to do without blaming others.

Apologize without allowing your regret or guilt to turn into embarrassment.

Accept responsibility for your actions and vow to make apologies.

Adopt an attitude of self-acceptance and faith in your own ability to improve.

Let your trusted friends and family know how you feel.

It's normal to feel uncomfortable when broaching the subject of personal guilt. Because admitting guilt is never simple. This means that feeling guilty can push you away from friends and family, which can make it harder to recover.

You may be concerned that others will look down on you because of what has occurred, but in most cases, this is not the case. In fact, you may find that friends and family provide invaluable assistance.

Your loved ones will likely be sympathetic and helpful. When people talk about their feelings, even negative or upsetting ones, it might help reduce stress.

When friends and relatives share their stories, it can make you feel like you're not alone. Just about everyone has done something they later came to regret, thus most individuals have experienced the pangs of remorse that accompany acknowledging wrongdoing.

Surviving guilt or guilt for an event over which you had no say can be alleviated with the help of an objective third party's viewpoint.

Chapter 10

CHANGE OF HEART AND HOPE

Lastly, we'll think about the Creator's eighth and last suggestion: have faith in God and have faith in the future. Is there no faith that God will intervene? Is there any truth to the claim that those who profess religion reap its benefits?

Having trust in God has been shown to lower stress levels, which in turn eliminates nerve-overvoltage and slows the rate at which telomeres shorten in cells. Telomeres are the biological clock of a cell. Each cell division causes them to shrink in size. disappear, causing the cells to die and the organ as a whole to perish. This explains why believers tend to live an extra 7-11 years than the general population.

RISING WITH OPTIMISM

Since hope influences so many facets of our lives, it's imperative that we figure out how to cultivate and sustain it. take heed to the advice provided below, which can restore faith.

Don't let hope fade from your mind. Worried about the future? Attempt to maintain an optimistic outlook. It's all about how you frame things in the outset. Relive happy moments and reflect on the positive aftereffects they had.

Conquer your mind of negative ideas. Negative New Year's Eve (nye) thinking is rife with fallacies that need to be exposed. Helps with both the act of quitting and the mental process of doing so. You shouldn't assume that just because something hasn't worked for you before that it can't work in the future. We need to identify the root causes of these setbacks, fix them, and then return command of the situation To put it another way, you shouldn't be enslaved by your history. Have no regrets about your previous lives. We tend to recall happy memories experiences and value the wisdom gained from them. If you focus on the good times from your past, you can look ahead to the future without dread.

Alter your own life's mundane routine. A person who is paralyzed by yearning and sadness might consider altering some aspect of their way of life. Get out of your comfort zone and experience something brand new, whether it's a new location, activity, friend you haven't seen in years, or kind of music. And if you haven't already, perhaps now is the time to delve into the wealth of knowledge contained in the Bible. These alterations will have an optimistic effect on your mental outlook for the future.

ACQUIRE A POSITIVE OUTLOOK ON LIFE THE TRIAL OF OPTIMISM AND HOPE

Nonetheless related. There are many competing explanations for the same event; consider the following examples: 1) "What if this head pain was actually caused by a brain tumor?" or: 2) "I'm sure this headache will go away soon." No diagnosis is complete without reading the revised thoughts. Every circumstance has both good and bad aspects that must be considered after gathering as much data as feasible. Nonetheless, I must refocus my attention on the good worry and good permission even, seemed would, seven days a week conditions.

BE ENCOURAGED FOR GOD IS LISTENING

God has made a path for those who have strayed from him in the past to find him again. And not just entry; there's plenty of camaraderie, too! One who has had their hearts renewed by Christ recognizes their complete helplessness apart from God's grace, understands the depths and ugliness of their sin, and realizes they have nothing to offer. As a result of Christ's sacrifice, Christians have hope that God will hear their prayers and grant them peace. The believer's life is always being nourished by the gushing stream of God's presence. Because of this, we know we are not helpless.

THE FACT THAT GOD IS MERCIFUL GIVES YOU REASON TO HAVE FAITH

In this verse, the vocalist admits his own sinfulness, which is a great assistance to the listener. He recognizes God's majesty and, consequently, realizes that he is helpless in the face of a holy God unless God makes a path for him. For all of God's faithful, God has. He has shown grace toward Christians by directing his righteous wrath upon Christ instead of us. Because of what Christ has done for us, God now considers us righteous and that gives us hope. Because of Christ, we are no longer under condemnation, even when our fleshly natures and our own consciences speak harshly against us.

HAVE FAITH BECAUSE GOD IS COMMUNICATING WITH YOU

The Bible is a miracle because it is God's living, active Word! During trying circumstances, you can find comfort in the knowledge that God has not abandoned you. God has made it possible for you to learn the truth and be purified by it. The Word of God is the Christian's sword in the spiritual battle that lies ahead. Trust that God will provide what you need to sustain a healthy, prosperous life in this moment.

BELIEVE THAT GOD WILL EVENTUALLY COME BACK FOR YOU

A watchman, literally "one who keeps watch," would stand guard over a certain area from a fortified wall in ancient times. They were paid to keep an eye out for invaders. Believers look forward to the "dawn," or the second coming of Christ when He will appear in tremendous grandeur and splendor from the skies above to usher in the creation of a brand new universe.

The Psalm exhorts us to keep our eyes on the present, to not give in to discouragement, and to resist the temptation to let the cares of the world take our focus away from what really matters. Being vigilant against the sinful influence in the world and in our own hearts is an essential part of the waiting process. As Christians, our faith is based on the certain knowledge that Christ will one day return in glory. It will happen, as certain and predictable as the sunrise.

BELIEVE THAT GOD WILL COMPLETE THE GOOD WORK HE HAS STARTED IN YOU

Confronting sin and realizing that we are aliens in this world can be depressing. However, Christians put their faith in God to bring their sanctification, or spiritual maturity, to fruition. While the sinner faces discouragement and hopelessness, the new creation has faith in the Holy Spirit's ability to produce fruit and activate good deeds. The Christian will be honored in the end, and this world is not our last destination.

INDEX